Angela Kilmartin was born in Essex. On leaving school she worked as a fashion model for some years and then studied at the Guildhall School of Music and Drama on singing and acting scholarships. In 1966 she married, and started disabling attacks of cystitis, complicated by thrush caused by continuous antibiotics. Five years later cystitis had put an end to her promising singing career and created tremendous difficulties in her marriage.

Then one urologist introduced her to self-help and a dramatic return to health. Angered by the lack of this simple advice over her five years of cystitis, Angela founded the famous U and I Club in 1971, a registered charity for teaching prevention and management of urinary problems to both patients and doctors. By 1980 both her books were available worldwide and the U and I Club was stopped.

The acknowledged authority on self-help in cystitis, she has, among other efforts, toured the USA for television and radio shows, lectured worldwide, made films, and instigated the Health Education Council leaflet on cystitis.

Angela has now returned to live in London after following her husband on postings to Nigeria and Saudi Arabia. She lectures and counsels on cystitis and enjoys solo oratorio work with choral societies around the country.

Also in Arrow by Angela Kilmartin

Understanding Cystitis – A Complete Self-Help Guide

VICTIMS OF THRUSH AND CYSTITIS

Angela Kilmartin

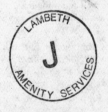
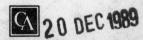
20 DEC 1989

Century Arrow
London Melbourne Auckland Johannesburg

A Century Arrow Book
published by Arrow Books Ltd
62–65 Chandos Place, London WC2N 4NW

An imprint of Century Hutchinson Ltd

London Melbourne Sydney Auckland
Johannesburg and agencies throughout
the world

First published in Great Britain 1986

Photoset in Linotron Ehrhardt by
Rowland Phototypesetting Limited
Bury St Edmunds, Suffolk

Printed and bound in Great Britain by
Guernsey Press Co. Ltd, Guernsey, C.I.

ISBN 0 09 940660 8

Contents

This book is dedicated to common sense. It is also dedicated to Mr John Wickham, FRCS, consultant urologist, who saw the need for common sense

PART ONE

CYSTITIS AND THRUSH

CHAPTER ONE

Angela

To put it simply, this new book is not so much about cystitis and thrush as about the victims of these hateful conditions.

'Can I join the U&I Club and could you tell me where my nearest branch is?'

'I'm afraid that you can't join the U&I Club because it closed in 1981 and in any case it never had branches because I, as founder, never allowed or encouraged them.'

These questions and my answers appear daily on my desk. Women want to meet other women with the same problem. The trouble is that it isn't the identical problem. Each case of cystitis and thrush is so different that what works for one woman won't always work for her neighbour and might even be harmful.

Perhaps, for any readers new to my work and books on these subjects, I should begin with further explanations.

In 1964, as a girl of twenty-two, I fell in love, and in 1966 we married. It was a lovely day, a lovely church, a lovely reception and we were a lovely couple. We did very little loving on our honeymoon, to say the least – it was utterly wrecked by honeymoon cystitis, the bride's disease!

From the third day, I was in severe pain, passing fresh running blood in my urine and pretty well comatose. My husband half-carried me into the en-suite bathroom and I sat on the lavatory screaming into a handkerchief to deaden the sound. I was incontinent – an exceptionally embarrassing experience for anyone, anywhere, anytime, let alone in a foreign country with a new young husband watching it all. I didn't know what the hell was going on because nothing like it had ever happened to me before in my life.

A woman doctor saw me and, in French, diagnosed *la cystite*! She prescribed a blue antiseptic pill; a large injection of penicillin into the buttocks each day for seven days; no further sex; no further swimming; no more alcohol and no more spicy food. I am still affected by this memory.

It was a waste; a devastation of all the thrill which we had hoped for and expected from our first-ever holiday together; a lastingly ghastly memory about happiness turning into horror. A honeymoon is the one holiday that cannot be repeated, and future holidays were similarly marred.

Not just holidays either, for over the next few years I was to have attacks of cystitis every three to four weeks. There was blood in the urine within hours, incontinence, and pain that made me crawl on the floor from bed to lavatory and back again. Fear came as well: fear of further future attacks and fear at the onset of the familiar first twinges. I came to know what it meant to cry *in* pain and to cry *out of* frustration.

Confidently at first, through 1966 and 1967, I put myself in the hands of the medical profession – where else? I visited my National Health Service GP, who still holds those early notes (we had a little smile about them only the other day), a private doctor just off Harley Street who is now, alas, dead, and St Bartholomew's Hospital urology out-patients' department.

Urine was usually tested and mostly found to have bacteria, which meant that antibiotics were prescribed. By 1967, I was being put on three months' worth at a time 'to kill the germs, dear'. There was an assortment on offer – sulphonamides, Ampicillin, tetracyclins, Furadantin, etc. These produced lethargy so severe after a lengthy course that my body simply could not live a normal day. Some mornings, it was only possible to reach the bathroom before being very pleased to stagger back to bed. I never had nausea and diarrhoea, only lethargy.

My first kidney X-ray, called an IVP (intravenous pyelogram) was, I think, taken at St Bartholomew's Hospital in London. This X-ray showed my kidneys to be clear but my bladder had signs of inflammation. More antibiotics were prescribed and I was returned to the care of my general practitioner.

So, additionally, I turned to private medicine. The private doctor near Harley Street decided to take me in for an overnight stay in a nursing convent for a cystoscopy. I was given a general anaesthetic and the doctor was then able to insert an instrument called a cystoscope right up into my bladder. He had a good look round and found absolutely nothing wrong, nothing there to worry about. Wonderful! I somehow didn't feel like celebrating, especially when I tried passing urine for the first time after the operation.

Another year went by, and it was suggested by a medical friend of mine that, having seen several doctors concerned specifically with the kidneys and bladder, I might try a gynaecologist. Nothing to be lost – so I went. The gynaecologist said straight out that cystitis was for urologists not gynaecologists, but he had heard that forgoing sex could be helpful to some women. Six months, he reckoned, I could try going without sex. Well, a sex life with my particular problems recurring every three or four weeks could not be called a sex life anyway! I was dreadfully sore and itchy, terrified by now of the pain, weariness, incontinence and diminished quality of life, so if six months without any sex at all was the answer, we'd certainly give it a go.

The six months produced three attacks and the end of the six months confirmed my worst fears that it hadn't worked.

You won't – well, you might – believe what the medical profession suggested next. Six months of antibiotics to run concurrently with no sex! I was still green as green; and I did it. Can you imagine where our lovely marriage was going? It was steering into a force ten gale with Beachy Head not a million miles away.

Did it work? Like hell it did!

I was pulled into hospital for two days for another full IVP and cystoscopy. Pain, tears and ALL CLEAR.

More cystitis. It had, I repeat, been happening every three to four weeks throughout all this time except during my first pregnancy, August 1968 to May 1969. So I had had nine months off. Treatment with antibiotics continued.

1970, and the private doctor says: 'I'll perform a cautery.' Cauterization meant burning away the outer layer of skin in the urethra – that's the little tube that carries urine out of the bladder to the opening. 'This,' he continued, 'will burn out all the infected skin and you will never again have cystitis.'

Wonderful! Wonderful! I was only amazed that it hadn't been done sooner; so much suffering could have been saved. Within a few days I was back in the convent nursing home like a lamb to the slaughter, still so innocent. The pain of trying to pass the first drops of concentrated post-operative urine took my breath away and made me stop.

The nuns started me on orange squash, and the inevitable moment arrived. One nun stood in the doorway, another held my head and pressed my screaming mouth into her uniform, and I writhed on that lavatory as I had never done before or since.

Five weeks of recovery passed before my husband and I began to put together some gentle sex over a few days. Sex was comfortable and well lubricated and I had not the slightest intention of lining it up as the cause of cystitis. Besides, no one had ever suggested a direct involvement. I had also had the pregnancy with sex and no cystitis plus the two periods of forbidden sex *with* cystitis, so where did that leave us? With a real conundrum.

Four days later, at dawn, the first signs of an attack began. My husband went to work at seven-thirty and I went out into the back garden carrying my wedding dress and going-away outfit. I was so deeply distressed that I had got to thinking the whole thing was being jinxed. The dustman came at nine o'clock and carried the jinx away. I can still see him walking past the roses with the bin on his back.

I made a cup of tea and went into the sitting room. There, with tears streaming down my cheeks, I closed the piano lid and shut out all lingering hopes of my excellent voice and acting talents ever finding fruition. That piano lid stayed down for seven years, nor would I, during those years, listen to radio concerts or visit concert or opera houses.

God, his marriage sacraments and his given gifts were, from now, finished with.

I returned to the kitchen and laundered some 'smalls'. My neighbour, a pleasant woman, hanging out her own washing early, remarked that I was an unusual sight in the garden at such a time. I told her of the latest signs of an attack.

'Well,' she said, 'after all you've been through, you're just going to have to learn to live with it.'

I didn't shout at her, I smiled – and walked back, pleading the need for the lavatory. I picked up a new bottle of two hundred codeine pills. I scarcely put it down all day except to see to my toddler. Didn't my neighbour realize that it was not humanly possible to live with such torment? The pain, the fear of more attacks, the awful incontinence, the loss of daily life and the loss of the comfort of marriage.

The terrible journey between bed and lavatory began again for the sixty-second time, roughly, since my wedding day. But I was now bordering on suicide. When you are newly suicidal you have an instinct to find someone to solve your problem. No one that I knew from the past five years was able to help. Where could I turn? The very practicality of doing away with cystitis still stabbed at my brain. If cystitis were to go, all the other problems would naturally follow. Where could I turn?

Believe it or believe it not, but I picked up the *Yellow Pages*. Towards the back was a section on urologists. Starting at the letter *A*, I rang every one of them to see if an appointment could be made for that day because at the end of that day, I had promised myself all the codeine. At *S*, one man had just had a 5 p.m. appointment cancelled, and by dint of my desperation, his secretary agreed to fit me in.

His consulting rooms in Harley Street were pale green and the three leather chairs were dark bottle-green. Everything was cool and calm. Ice-stiff and desperate, without make-up to show my puffy eyes, I sat there explaining.

He examined me and announced that there was some swelling and redness caused obviously by today's attack. He asked about past urine samples and I replied that I thought I had had something called E.Coli plus pus cells and things on several occasions. We also discussed sex and I said that I was sure this couldn't be involved because there had been countless attacks when sex had been no-where in sight.

The urologist sat back, pushed away the folder and said, 'I am not going to give you any further treatment nor am I even going to write you a prescription for antibiotics for this attack. Instead, I am going to tell you to do something. Pass water after intercourse and drink plenty of fluid when an attack starts.'

If it's possible to sob, smile and smirk at the same time, then that is what I did. Then I blurted out, 'I have come to you in rock bottom, suicidal desperation *and* paid ten guineas. I want pills not a sentence. I want the latest drug, the latest research, the latest medical advance.'

'There is none, Mrs Kilmartin. You have had everything, and

more, that the medical profession can offer. Why not just try passing water after intercourse? It seems to work well in sexually active women. My next patient coming in for a check-up tried it and after thirty-two years of cystitis, she's free of it and her husband comes home for lunch and sex every day to make up for those lost years!'

In my mind, I swore. Never could a mere sentence of advice turn round my marriage, my singing career and my life quality from the awful trauma of the last four and a half years – never! I did not believe him, and left. He had reckoned that a month would show me if his advice was likely to be going to work.

At home, I told my husband of the day, of the medical explanation about E.Coli and sex given by the urologist. We had a long discussion on the state of the marriage because it had taken a real battering through absolutely no fault of our own, and reckoned that by pulling our sex life round, the ensuing closeness would make the superficial tensions dissolve. We made an appointment with each other to try intercourse a week later, after this current attack had subsided (with antibiotics from the NHS doctor).

I tried out having sex and passing water afterwards several times that month – no cystitis! Breathing heavily, we started on the second month and nearly made it before another attack began. I did, however, see the reasoning behind the urologist's idea and felt that it had proven itself sufficiently to adopt it. Outside my one pregnancy, this period of time was the longest without cystitis in our marriage – now five years old.

All during these years, I had also suffered bouts of uncontrollable irritation in my bowels and around the vaginal orifice. Once or twice only had my doctor looked in the vagina and found thrush. Usually, out of great ignorance, I never mentioned the irritation. The times when I did were when I had woken up in the middle of the night scratching so hard that I bled. My husband used to wake up, too! Don't forget, reader, that there was no mention on radio or TV or in the press, even the women's press, about such indelicate matters – absolutely taboo subjects, they were. Three out of the five years of cystitis so far, I had had rampant thrush to contend with and muddle everything, but I was very raw in every sense of the word about how and why.

On this special attack after seven weeks' remission, a vaginal examination took place. It showed thrush, and the urine sample was clear: no urinary infection. So the private doctor treated the thrush with pessaries and Nystatin tablets, and I drank a great deal of water to help the urinary discomfort. Ten days later he did a thrush clearance check and I was all right.

At this point, I am going to say that similar patches of remission occurred and thrush also occurred over the whole of the next year. I was by no means one hundred per cent cleared of cystitis, and because I couldn't learn about thrush from any one source, I put my knowledge together slowly. In fact, those five years of antibiotic treatment left my system and my perineum very prone to vaginitis, particularly thrush, for many years – and it is still weak to this day.

What was coming to me in intensifying brilliance was the thought that someone had shown me that I, Angela, could beneficially help myself a little. Just passing urine after intercourse is helping yourself – self-help. A doctor can't pass urine for you, you must do it yourself.

'Learn to live with it,' my neighbour had said. Self-help *is* learning to live with it, but from the optimistic and positive viewpoint of routing it, beating it. I had only ever taken the defeatist, pessimistic viewpoint of 'putting up with it', letting and expecting the doctor to do all the work.

Was there anything else, perhaps, that I could gainfully do to help myself to beat it? By God, there was as much burning hatred in my soul for cystitis as there had ever been burning urine in my bladder – my marriage nearly gone, my singing career completely abandoned. You can't sing when you're unhappy and heavily drugged, so I was now swearing instead. And I swore to myself that as long as I lived, the urologist's simple sentence of advice was going to be available somehow to any and all of the countless women in Great Britain who, as I now knew, were also in the same boat as myself.

What I didn't have the foggiest idea about, as yet, were the vagaries and intricacies and varieties of this bladder condition called cystitis.

I didn't yet know that symptoms like mine were not necessarily identical in every sufferer; that doctors called almost anything to do with the bladder cystitis; that urine was not always infected; and that there were lots of causes.

I didn't know because I didn't need to know; I didn't know because I'd never talked to another sufferer; I didn't know because

I was not medically minded, trained or the least bit interested. I did want to get well, though.

My previous life had been glamorous and artistic – no interest at all in swabs and sluices. I now had a baby daughter and a husband, who tended to keep me busy with meals, walks and shopping. My whole married life so far had been a nightmare of unwanted pain and frustration, and with this new light possibly shining from the end of a five-year tunnel, there was much to think about apart from dwelling on illness.

What seared my brain most was the persistent thought that I'd paid ten guineas, a lot of money in 1970, to be given a sentence of words that made my condition show an improvement. Why on earth hadn't one of the many doctors known it or told me it?

Did they know it? If not, why not? Weren't they taught it at medical school, or was it considered beneath them? Heavens above, was it because they were men? I truly couldn't believe that. A doctor was sworn on oath to help the sick and save life, wasn't he?

The medical profession had unloaded hundreds of hours and hundreds of pounds in attempting to treat my cystitis successfully. I'd also spent hundreds of pounds within the private sector, not to mention the hundreds of hours of suffering. No, it couldn't be because they were men – if they could have got rid of this pestering patient, they surely would have done so.

I was left facing the distinct possibility that indeed they didn't know about passing water after intercourse.

St Bartholomew's Hospital in the City of London received a letter from me addressed to the senior consultant urologist.

CHAPTER TWO

The U&I Club

He sent me this reply:

Dear Madam,
  Thank you very much for your full and interesting letter and your suggestions with regard to the development of some sort of collective action to combat this problem of urinary tract infection in women. I have taken the liberty of discussing your letter with my colleagues. They feel, as I do myself, that probably the first step would be to meet you and discuss some of the problems of this condition as they appear to us from the medical side and then try to work out how we would best cooperate for the benefit of the many women afflicted by this disease.
  I would suggest that the best thing you could do would be to come to St Bartholomew's Hospital on a Friday afternoon at about 4 o'clock to meet the consultants concerned during their normal weekly conference. Let me know when this would be convenient to you and we will all arrange to be there and discuss the matter.
  I would be very keen myself on some sort of news sheet as the more propaganda that we can get disseminated about this distressing condition and its management the better, and I have a few ideas myself. I think we could best dicuss them together rather than trying to communicate rather long windedly through the post.

At 3 o'clock on Friday, 1 January 1971, I got up from bed, where I had been dealing with another attack of cystitis, the first for three months. I dressed and drove to St Bartholomew's – ten minutes away.
  The waiting room in the urology unit out-patients' was virtually empty as the clock on the wall showed 4 o'clock. A passing nurse smiled at my name and showed me the door of the consultants'

office. I opened it and gaped. The senior consultant had meant what he said.

The room was full of doctors and nurses; two sat on a filing cabinet, others perched on any flat surface or stood around the twelve by sixteen foot floor space. I was welcomed and shown to a chair to sit beside the senior consultant. In a soft voice he briefly introduced me to Them and Them to me. Some more of Them drifted in as we began.

I asked why this unit, in two years of treating me for acute recurrent cystitis, had failed to tell me to pass water after intercourse. Many replies were offered and it seemed finally that they knew about it but hadn't the time to say it. Time was for them an unbeatable enemy.

'Why haven't you produced a small sheet of paper with it written down, plus anything else which you feel may be helpful to women like me? We can take it home to read. What other tips do you know but don't tell us about?'

'We have been thinking of writing just such a sheet but we haven't done anything about it yet. Liverpool Hospital has had a sheet of tips for cystitis sufferers handed out in its urology unit for the last year. I've got a copy here.'

'It seems,' I said a little later, 'that with such vast numbers of women cystitis sufferers, not a lot is being done for them. Is it because' – and I swallowed – 'we are women? If men suffered in the same numbers, would more progress towards a cure be made?'

A registrar remonstrated quickly. 'I've just written a book on urinary problems and I've done a whole chapter on women – a whole chapter!'

I breathed in and responded, 'Is that all?'

There was silence.

We began to look forward to implementing more help for women coming to this unit. A similar leaflet to Liverpool Hospital's was discussed, and then I wondered. I wondered aloud why only these highly localized patients should be helped. Why not try to help on a national level? Hundreds of thousands of women all over the country were afflicted, and their doctors were impotent in helping them effect lasting relief from attacks.

Who suggested it I can't remember, but shortly, I found a deal being struck between Them and me. If I did the organizing and thought of a way to distribute it, They would help medically in any necessary way to publish a newsletter for sufferers. With bi-monthly printing of advice, updates and additions could be made – and it would provide the women themselves with the opportunity to pass on tips which they might be finding helpful. Perhaps such a newsletter could form the basis for some sort of association.

I learned years later that They felt quite unconcerned over my ability to do all this, despite my never having done such a thing, but They were concerned that I might become affected and depressed at the numbers and the dreadful tales that I would undoubtedly start to hear. I did doubt my own unproven ability at organizing something prospectively so huge, but it certainly never entered my mind to become depressed about the numbers or the suffering.

There was so much hatred in my soul for cystitis – and so much love for my thwarted singing and husband – that I enjoined myself very eagerly into doing battle against it. Love and hate – the most ancient motivators known to man and I gave them both full rein.

The name 'The U&I Club' was conceived a few days after the meeting at St Bartholomew's. The bedside lights had been out for half an hour and my husband was already snoring lightly. The name came, and I sat up, switched on the lamp and reached for pencil and paper, proclaiming: 'I've got it, I've got it.'

My husband listened amazed – in fact, he'd had a pretty amazing few days of me anyway. So I explained:

> U&I for you and I
> U&I for urinary infection
> The U&I Club.

Not that my old English mistress would have been too happy with the grammar, but there we are! It was to become the only bladder charity in the world, renowned for its high membership levels, and for its pioneering work in this field of medicine.

It was not primarily founded for fund-raising or for scientific research. It was founded to educate the patient and her doctor to promote self-help. Later chroniclers have listed some of the reasons for my successful public relations work for the U&I Club. Doctors can be funny people and won't always listen to a patient, but over the years I have lectured to hundreds of them. They say that I'm a good public speaker, that I look nice and that I don't antagonize. I can promote controversy within the medical profession, and indeed do set out to stimulate broader ideas on cystitis. It has helped greatly to have a stage background so that interviews in the press and on TV and radio aren't traumatic or frightening, and I've achieved a name for persistency and honesty. What's more, I don't mind saying 'urine' out loud!

These attributes were vital weapons for my battle. The U&I Club applied for and received full charity status from the Charity Commissioners in London, but we all had a huge laugh at the legalities which finally categorized us as a 'fellowship'! On paper we were termed 'The U&I Fellowship'!

How on earth does one print and publish a newsletter nationwide?

It couldn't be sold in a shop, so it had to be mailed. Who would help me over the printing? A friend of my husband's edited an in-house business journal and kindly taught me the rudiments of choosing print types, designing the layout and instructing printers. He introduced me to the printers which his journal used, in Warley, Worcestershire. This family firm, Cradley Printing, printed countless items for me over the years, including a booklet, leaflets, magazines, cards, letterheads – anything. They also supplied the envelopes and had good warehousing for storage. A twice-weekly van to London gave me marvellous back-up service to my door. Nothing was ever late or impossible, and the eagerness to help of their drivers, telephonists and managers was an example to all industry. I was so lucky.

Where were my offices to be? They had to be at home because of my baby daughter. I started out on the dining table and then had to move upstairs to the small bedroom. This was fitted out with a custom-made desk and shelf unit. A local friend was part-time typist as required, for a bottle of wine!

Was I paid? No, but every one else was – by mutual agreements, and none proved greedy.

How did I decide on membership and office systems? Alice Neville, who ran the Agoraphobics so successfully in the 1960s, was a tower of information on the technicalities of running a club by post and starting on a system that would be able to cope with an increasing membership. Within three years we had to go on to a computer; I never realized how often the British change houses!

What of publicity? Indeed, what of it! I sat on the telephone for the best part of eighteen months to cover fully the national press, the women's press, the radio stations and the television. TV people were very sceptical, and finally in 1973 I was allowed a slot of forty minutes in the second series of *Open Door* produced by the Community Service Unit at the BBC. I still hold the response record because we stopped counting after the twelve thousandth letter. The flood just went on and on.

The early press and radio coverage deserves special mention. It was hard gained, but very successful in blowing down the doors of this highly taboo topic. Producers and interviewers were naturally very pleased with the tremendous reactions from their particular sections of the public and suddenly realized that here indeed was a new topic.

At first, though, the water was very rough. I was refused an advert placing in the London *Evening News* by the classified ads manager. He didn't like the word 'cystitis' or the seeking of women readers to become members. We bargained and settled for:

> Cystitis? Sufferers needing a
> sympathetic chat and tea, ring—

I had forty phone calls in two days, but only one woman turned up for the tea and sympathy. One of the phone calls was from a journalist working, he said, for *GP* magazine, which belonged to the Haymarket Publishing Group. I agreed to his request to come and interview me.

He came round that afternoon, but an hour later, when he had spent most of the time talking about masturbation, I showed him the door and telephoned his supposed employers. They denied all knowledge of this person – and I knew I'd been tricked. However, *GP* magazine liked my spiel on cystitis and sent a real reporter to do the first medical magazine interview with me on the new U&I Club.

Some months later, the man who took my call about the bogus journalist rang me from me his new job on *The Sunday Times*. He was Oliver Gillie, the intrepid health research journalist, who proceeded to give the U&I Club its first national newspaper write-up in *The Sunday Times* for November 1971.

The first women's magazine item was a one-inch notification of our founding together with the address in *She*.

Whilst all this was developing, a friend rang and said that *Woman's Hour* on BBC radio had just mentioned cystitis in a listeners' query session. Why didn't I ring them about the new club?

I rang. The six-week-old postmen's strike had effectively stopped *Woman's Hour* letters from listeners. This meant that I could give a short telephone letter of notification but not an address. So the next day at 3 p.m. it was read out over the air and my phone number was given, with my approval.

My phone rang instantly and I didn't manage to put it down until 11.30! It began again at 9 a.m. the next morning and continued all day. My daughter had to go to a neighbour. *Woman's Hour* was similarly affected, and I was invited on the programme three weeks and hundreds of phone calls later to explain myself for twenty minutes. It was my first-ever proper radio interview and I was very grateful to be able to remember a few helpful tips from my old Guildhall drama course, which had included some training in microphone technique. The post which arrived after the postal strike ended was enough to put fear into my heart. Even my mother came up to help open the envelopes.

Because of this one programme, the U&I Club's first edition in May 1971 of its highly vetted magazine went out to over 200 women up and down the country. *The Sunday Times'* half-page article in November doubled our December edition. The snowball had begun to roll.

The magazine had a format:

Cover page A proverb or saying to give hope. Editor's comment

Pages 2, 3, 4 Ideas and tips from members (did *they* teach us!) Letters from members and doctors

Page 5 Case histories

Page 6 General article related in some way to the subject

Page 7 Questioner's Forum – medically answered queries

Page 8 A medical article written by a doctor

The print size decreased rapidly to accommodate incoming items whilst retaining the same eight pages. We used photographs and diagrams and very high-quality glossy paper. It was foolscap size – large by today's standards of newsletters.

The professional press stood amazed at our ability to fill such a magazine every two months on one topic, and I was reported as saying that 'we could double the size but I don't want to run the risk of boring them out of belonging to the club'. There was no chance of that. Membership two years later, in May 1973, was eight thousand for any one month, computerized and climbing!

The small bedroom had quickly become hopelessly inadequate, so my husband and I moved to a four-storey house. Here I had my second child – a boy – and the basement for U&I offices. The membership fee had begun at one pound a year, including post and packing. All costs were covered, but I refused to work to a profit, saying that these women had already given, like myself, in time, money and suffering. We should not demand a penny more from them than the costs. We never did.

The tips from members were medically discussed and experimented with on my own still-suffering (but not so frequently) body. Hygiene measures were begun and adapted; dealing with an attack of cystitis in the middle of the night was defined, refined and printed in every edition; liquid intake and diet became a popular aspect of prevention. And so we – the patients and doctors – slowly and so carefully, documented for the first time those tips for prevention and management of cystitis that have proved the salvation of marriages, family life, jobs and sanity ever since.

It was a remarkable effort and a highly successful campaign for nine years. It took on the taboo and beat its own ignorance.

My last ever – and it was a bolt out of the blue – attack of cystitis took place in a caravan in France in August 1976. I'd overdone the French wine and the twice-daily holiday sex! I managed the attack myself with water-drinking, painkillers and bicarbonate of soda – no pills, no doctor, no fear. I have not had a single attack since that day, because I prevent it every day of my life, just as I prevent tooth decay by cleaning my teeth.

My many scrapbooks are filled with press cuttings, my memories are of eighteen-hour days concerned with all sorts of activities and publicity: radio programmes, TV programmes (because the professionals watched that 1973 *Open Door* programme and decided that the subject had a proven viewer response), film-making, book-writing (this book is my fourth), magazine articles, lecturing to doctors and to women's groups all over the country, helping drug companies on varying research, the riveting fascination of one-to-one counselling – and of those huge vehicle-delivered mailbags arriving every day packed with letters from all over the world. In 1975 my post was twenty thousand letters with members in forty-six countries. I had two full-time secretaries, plus myself, and twelve part-time envelope-packers.

The oil sheikhs caused a twenty-six per cent rise in inflation in 1975 and I could no longer cost the membership fee from one edition to the next. The magazine had to go. Under great pressure to continue, I still went ahead with writing a fifty-page booklet called *Self-help in Cystitis*, and between 1975 and 1981 we must have distributed 80–100,000 copies just through the U&I Club's office in my home.

The oil sheikhs also wrecked my husband's costings in a building venture in which he was involved. He lost a lot of money and decided to go to Nigeria with his main work. I remained in England and was forced to sell the big house. It was six months before pressures eased and the children and I could obtain a visa to visit Lagos.

Thus commenced six years of his working abroad. I was torn between being a wife, a mother, a campaigner. The decision which I finally had to take meant putting husband and marriage first, then children, and cystitis third. So I wrote my third book *Cystitis – the Complete Self-Help Guide* and promoted it heavily both in the UK and in the States, where I had sold the manuscript myself, and prayed that women would in future look in the bookshops for help with cystitis and thrush.

In 1980, the U&I Club regretfully closed, although the post, much lessened now by my absences abroad affecting publicity, still came and still comes. In 1982 my husband returned to work in England and we set up home in London. The pressures on us from his involvement in travel and work have brought about a very sad divorce, and in the aftermath of that, I have once again turned to writing and counselling. I have also started singing again and enjoy solo work with choral societies.

It seems that I have come round in a circle whilst continuing to keep to the vow that I made, which was never to let another woman suffer ignorantly from cystitis. Doctors and their patients are now both aware that it is possible to prevent cystitis, and the main campaigning has been responsible for this.

The next chapter is a scaled-down self-help guide intended for those women who have not read any of my previous books. For those who have read the others, regard this as a recap of the main points before you settle in to the case histories which form this fourth book.

CHAPTER THREE

Cystitis

The name derives from the Greek '*cyst*', meaning a sac or a pouch
– hence bladder, and '*itis*', meaning inflammation.

    urethritis means inflammation of the urethra

    trigonitis means inflammation of the trigone

    vaginitis means inflammation of the vagina

Cystitis is a symptom of one or several background health conditions.
To stop further attacks of cystitis you must find and remedy these
other conditions, or 'causes', as I like to call them.

Until 1971 doctors and patients, through lack of information,
dealt only with the attack itself. They frequently and unfortunately
still have this same old blinkered approach. The essence of my work
over the years has been to promote the existence and the subsequent
prevention and management of those causes. Some are very obvious,
others downright obscure, but eighty per cent of them occur because
of the lifestyle of the modern patient and her family.

We have thought of cystitis as being a condition on its own. It's
easy enough to think this way because cystitis has its own set of
symptoms. They are:

PAIN when you pass water.

FREQUENCY when you need to pass urine a lot.

BLEEDING from the urethra whilst passing water.

During a consultation with your doctor you don't always ask what's
causing this, you usually expect him to clear up these three nasty
symptoms quickly. Once they have gone you think it's gone for good
and you're cured. I never use the word 'cure' when talking or writing
about cystitis. 'Cure' conjures up the idea it will never come back.
That's fallacious. It's only gone until the next time! Next time will
come again and again for many women until they find the cause or

causes of their own brand of cystitis. Some of you may be thinking after this that you don't have true cystitis. Perhaps you never bleed but still have the other two symptoms. There are several variations:
    frequency only,
    backache and low pelvic ache
    high temperature and general malaise
    urethral stinging
    sensations in the urethra
    or any combinations of these
Perhaps your doctor, on hearing you mention 'trouble with my waterworks', doesn't take an in-depth symptom list and saves time by calling it cystitis and writing a quick prescription.

Most bladder infections or inflammations start on the outside – the perineum, which is the name given to what lay people describe as 'my bottom'. It is also possible for an infection affecting, say, your lungs, to be severe enough to spread into the bloodstream and affect the kidneys' output of urine, which in turn dictates to the bladder that it is to empty at an increased rate.

The commonest cystitis, though, does travel upwards and inwards – reasons come later. Some types of bacteria can invade the vagina, but that doesn't become painful. The pain is situated in the highly delicate skin tissues of the urethra, which leads from the perineum into the bladder. Once the skin in the urethra has started to be attacked by the invading inflammation/infection, it tingles. These 'tingles' or 'sensations' worsen and set up a reaction from the bladder to empty itself. The urine flows down the urethra and washes over the tingling urethral skin. Urine is normally mildly acidic under everyday circumstances, dependent on what you have been drinking and how much.

If the invasion up the urethra continues, the tingling becomes an actual pain, and with every further act of micturition (passing of water) the relativity between pain and frequency gets closer. Each act of micturition leaves the bladder empty, and with a steadily ascending inflammation/infection, the end of the 2.5 centimetre-long urethra is reached. Entry into the bladder itself happens next.

The bladder skin reacts to the invasion by increasing the urge to empty and rid itself of the trouble. It almost seems to want to push itself down. 'Bearing down' is a phrase much used by cystitis victims to describe this particular sensation – it's a dragging, burning feeling and the pelvic area aches, too.

Within a short time there seems to be, and is, a long length of internal burning or knife-like pain, often quite excruciating.

The kidneys have to react to all this by producing more urine for the bladder to excrete, so they become 'excited'. They produce larger amounts of uric acid – this is the real burner – but have less and less body water with which to dilute it. The invasion is still ever upward, don't forget, so once out of the bladder it starts to progress up each of the two ureters. The ureters are fine spaghetti-like tubes, each one leading into a kidney. The downward flow of urine into the bladder is controlled in each ureter by a one-way sphincter valve – clever stuff! Each valve opens on response to gathered droplets of urine and closes after the urine has passed through. I once saw this happen during a cystoscopy that I was privileged to be allowed to view – very thrilling – to look into a body and watch it at work.

The invasion of the kidneys is called pyelitis, and now you will really get the backache and feel unwell. Shivers run throughout the body and you're pretty well bedbound by this stage. You're in one hell of a shivery, painful and embarrassed mess.

If you've had several attacks you will also know fear, tension and frustration. If you've had lots of attacks you will know marital trouble, inability to hold a job and severe depression. At this stage, if you are unlucky enough to have a ghastly doctor, he will probably say that you are neurotic and stick you on tranquillizers – DON'T LET HIM.

The life quality of a regular cystitis victim is sadly seldom assessed by the medical profession. They only assess the possible aspect of kidney scarring – you're not going to die of cystitis, because a course of antibiotics will 'stop the rot'!

So we're dealing with a condition that is exceptionally common, easy enough on the surface for the GP to treat, variable in symptoms, and which causes much upheaval and suffering.

If it's possible to think back in time before antibiotics, before even the earliest sulpha drugs – what did women take when they got cystitis? How did they deal with it and who told them? Now don't bombard me with homoeopathic and naturist 'cures', it's the principle that I'm interested in.

As for any thought of causes, I'm sure that women only had very vague ideas of them. 'Brides' disease' was obvious because sexual intercourse began on marriage, usually. Of course, it is still one of today's causes, except that I now term it 'onset of regular sexual relations'.

I doubt whether hygiene would have occurred to anyone, because water was carefully looked after and not on tap. Homes were too cold to bare much skin, and privacy for washing was scarce. The village whore might well have offered a bowl of water and a cloth to ward off 'the clap'. Can you imagine the same bowl, water and cloth all evening!

Way back, they had none of the promotional lifestyle causes that you will shortly read about, and life for many women was an existence governed by multiples of nine months, and often short. Mistresses were there in plenty later on, so presumably they of all women cared about how they smelt and how often they would need to be available and well.

If the average woman in the past was unaware of causes, would this mean that cystitis was not such a common problem as now? Communication between women was chatty and daughter learnt from mother. There were no newspapers, books or magazines – and even in 1966 no one wrote about cystitis in the existing journals, I can tell you!

Perhaps the women had words between them in the language that implied and described cystitis without requiring a deeper knowledge. Perhaps it came under the heading of folk medicine – folklore.

The treatments used during an attack would have been local to the area, but most people had to live near a supply of running water and this would have formed the basis of their treatment. Local herbs and vegetation supplied by those early witchdoctors, brave outcasts and often women, would have been boiled and infused with water. I'll bet a lot of the vegetation potions didn't taste nice or even work, but what would have worked – and still does – was the *amount* of water in the brew.

If there was no running water, as in the desert areas of countries like India and Africa, women would turn to something like coconuts or watermelons – bland, sterile, liquid-containing objects formed by other forces in nature.

Certain infections, specifically that called E.Coli, will after three or four days apparently burn themselves out. E.Coli will multiply by itself every 12.5 minutes, and if after a severe attack all the healthy skin layers in the urinary tract and kidneys have been invaded, there is little else for it to thrive on. The kidneys would bear scar tissues that, untreated, would render them finally unable to function. Thus, centuries ago, death was the ultimate release from suffering.

So you would have visited the witch, learnt from Mother or suffered in untreated silence.

How much of this can we use? There is no doubt that modern medical treatment is very much the baby in so far as centuries of home treatment history goes. Have we found that modern antibiotic treatment works?

Modern use of antibiotics has, in just ten years, been heavily revised. In the late 1960s and early 1970s, a ten to fourteen days' course was insisted on. Depending upon the drug, you need now only take antibiotics for five to seven days, and one drug company has a three-day course. The side-effects of such lengthy courses proved problematical for continuing victims of cystitis who required several courses of treatment in any one year. Diarrhoea, nausea, vomiting, lethargy and monilia (thrush), from the antiobiotics, caused as much suffering as the cystitis itself.

In an effort to stop this, dosages were reduced until they dealt just as well with the bacteria (if any were found) but decreased the possibility of side-effects. Newer types of antibiotics have also helped.

The action of antibiotics is to kill bacteria. All bacteria is killed by them – the good, the bad and the ugly! The unfortunate killing-off of the goodies is what gives rise to a thrush outbreak. The shorter the course, the less the risk and the quicker your body defences resume normal working.

So they do work – on that one attack! Ask yourself: Is that good? Is that all I want? Or do I want to stop future attacks?

ANTIBIOTICS won't stop future attacks.

ANTIBIOTICS are costly to our NHS.

ANTIBIOTICS on private prescription are costly to me.

ANTIBIOTICS still carry the risk of side-effects.

ANTIBIOTICS are usually given regardless of proven infection. An infection in the urine is proved present by a urine culture. This culture is made in laboratory conditions from a sample of your urine.

Not just any old sample. It must be from the first voidance of the day or from the start of an attack, when the bacterial count is at its highest, and before you start drinking.

Supposing the sample proves negative. See now what I meant by using two words to describe cystitis: inflammation/infection?

An attack of cystitis isn't *always* caused by bacteria. The next chapter will illustrate some non-bacterial cystitis but my other books, particularly *Cystitis – A Complete Self-Help Guide* will provide better detail. So if cystitis isn't always caused by bacteria, why take antibiotics?

Why indeed! Here the past centuries meet the twenty-first century. A combination of drinking and the use of antibiotics needs considering. Supposing that you and your doctor were to hold the antibiotics as a reserve treatment – to be used when the attack had got into the kidney *or* when a heavy bacterial count was found in the urine sample. Would that make sense? Yes of course. The best of the modern world still there to use, but only when absolutely essential.

Not all attacks of cystitis are bacterially monitored. Many is the tale that I could tell of doctors having a quick look to the light or flatly refusing to send the sample for culture. On first thought we would consider this bad doctoring, but there are other aspects:

It could turn out negative, which would mean an unnecessary drug intake and an unnecessary waste of money.

You're half-way through the course of pills before the result is known.

Any newly presenting patient with cystitis should have her first three attacks cultured. It's worth knowing, so that she knows, and can in future prevent, that particular kind of bacterial infection. It's also worth knowing if the results are negative, because she can concentrate on non-bacterial causes for preventive action.

With the antibiotics held in reserve, let's explore the earlier self-help of centuries back. In the previous slightly technical explanations of how the urinary tract works, we found that the burning in a cystitis attack is caused by concentrations of uric acid from the kidneys. The concentrated acid comes from:

kidney stimulus
bladder voidance
insufficient dilution

If we wish to reverse those three procedures we would decrease all stimulus by:

1 desensitizing the kidneys
2 alkalizing the uric acid
3 raising the amount of body liquid

This was the effect of the folk medicine used by women for many centuries. In 1971, I printed the following set of rules to be followed from the first twinges of an attack. It arose from medical and lay suggestions and was finally refined at St Bartholomew's after much discussion. It has been printed, copied and used by millions of women the world over. An early E.Coli bacterial attack will be flushed out and not require antibiotic treatment if the attack disappears. An attack unrelated to bacterial invasion will be eased. The routine will also show after three hours whether the attack has totally abated or whether your perineum still remains sore and twingy. Go to a VD, genito-urinary out-patients' or special clinic like Marie Stopes House for a full vaginal check with swabs. Possibly, unknown as yet to you, a vaginal problem is 'leaking' and upsetting the urethral orifice.

No matter what time the attack starts, react:

1 Take a urine specimen and store it in a container in the fridge until you can get it as soon as possible to a laboratory.
2 Drink half a pint of bland liquid now and every twenty minutes for three hours. Water mostly. Flavour it with a weak squash, not juice, sometimes.
3 On the hour every hour for three hours take: 1 level teaspoon of bicarbonate of soda to neutralize the acidity. Mix it in jam or take it in a small amount of liquid quickly, followed by a longer drink to take the taste away. Heart patients must discuss this with a doctor first. If for any reason you can't abide the bicarbonate have a go at Cymalon, which is a powder form of sodium citrate and acts similarly to the bicarb. This is manufactured by Sterling Health and available at all chemists without a prescription.
4 Take two or three strong painkillers at the start of the attack.
5 Fill two hot-water bottles – one to put at your back and the other well wrapped in a towel to put between the legs. This makes the urine feel cooler as it runs over the tingling perineal skin.
6 Once an hour for the three hours drink a COFFEE CUP of

strong coffee – no more no less. This acts to help you pass the large amount of water which is being drunk.

7 Put your feet up, read one of my other books on cystitis and try to find the reason for this attack.

The attack will diminish considerably if not totally disappear, and certainly the pain will go. You will know that your kidneys are free from bacterial damage and that you have avoided the alternative of antibiotics. After the three hours you may like to drink half a pint of water or very weak tea every one and a half hours just to retain the comfort level. If the soreness level starts to rise again and urethral twinges become distinct, go, as I said, for a full vaginal check straight away.

This, then, is true cystitis. Variations will be seen within the case histories of the rest of the book. The simple procedure of managing an attack removes the fear, pain and distress, aids the diagnosis, and saves money and time off work, whilst safeguarding the kidneys.

From the attack itself, we must move to some basic self-help prevention. It is obviously not possible to reproduce all the self-help that I have carefully set down in my other books, so I recommend *Understanding Cystitis and Cystitis – A Complete Self-Help Guide*, both now available in a new two-in-one cover from Arrow Books.

If you have never before read anything on cystitis and thrush and have found this book on a shelf somewhere, I should tell you some primary prevention. As each victim comes up in the book deeper explanations of my recommendations will be given.

Hygiene

The commonest bacterium known to cause urinary-tract infection is Escerischia Coliform – E.Coli. It lives in the bowel and if not confined internally will proceed along the perineum to the urethral orifice. It breeds in normal mildly acidic urine. To confine E.Coli to its normal habitat means having and maintaining an excellent daily hygiene procedure. It is not a matter of how often you wash but whether you are washing:

(a) properly
(b) after a bowel movement
(c) before or after intercourse as appropriate

The only way to wash the anal orifice properly after any kind of bowel movement is:

1 Use toilet tissue
2 Wash, rinse and resoap your hands
3 With a soapy hand cleanse the anal orifice (back passage)
4 *Don't* soap any other part of the perineum – EVER
5 Rinse your hands
6 Fill any old tonic/soda bottle with WARM water (not hot or cool)
7 Sit back on the lavatory and pour the water down your perineum, using the free hand to reach the nooks and crannies.
8 When all the soap has cleared, pat dry with a small towel or flannel
9 Never use a bidet or squat in the bath using the shower

This process MUST be done after every bowel movement every day of your life. Don't use cloths, flannels, cotton wool – only the clean flow of water from the bottle.

More information will occur later on and is already in the other books.

Sexual hygiene

1 Make sure that you and your partner have clean, trim fingernails.
2 Make sure that your partner can retract and clean the foreskin and, if circumcized, has a good standard of sexual cleanliness. (I once knew a German girl in America who swears she always insisted on a visual examination first!)
3 If you have washed after passing a stool (and you should anyway) a quick sluish of water from the bottle will just freshen the perineum. Should you not have removed faecal material then do so now as instructed. Don't ever have intercourse if faecal material is still present.
4 Don't indulge in rectal petting/intercourse.
5 Use KY Jelly as a buffer against bruising and dryness.
6 After intercourse, pass urine and pour cool water over the perineum as you sit on the lavatory. This will rinse off sexual liquids, which can go stale and cause irritation. It will also reduce inflammation from sexual buffeting.

Contraceptives

Hazardous! The only criterion is to find out which sort suits you (and your partner, though do think of yourself first, please; it is, after all, your body). Read any good book or literature, and always be prepared to change your contraceptive. In my life, I have used the sheath, spermicidal creams and tablets, the Pill, withdrawal and given my ex-husband a vasectomy for Christmas! I never tinkered with the cap or coil because of childbirth injuries and the lengthy cystitis history.

All contraceptives are capable of aggravating or causing cystitis in any given patient. If cystitis or thrush seemingly begins concurrent with starting any contraceptive, be watchful, wary and ready to stop using that method. Different times in a woman's life cycle may demand a different contraceptive to suit the circumstance.

Liquid intake

The yardstick for this is your own urinary comfort, not anyone else's. If your urine doesn't burn or tingle, is variable in colour, and you have no urinary problems, then whatever you are drinking is all right. Don't become dehydrated either in hot offices or on sunny beaches. Under such circumstances drink more plain water until you get the urinary colour and comfort back to what you consider normal.

Alcohol, strong coffee and strong tea will stimulate the kidneys. Don't overdo any of them and always be ready to drink a glass of water to dilute or sandwich such beverages.

Food intake

You would be amazed at some of the foods that people eat! Pounds of raspberries and strawberries because someone they know is an expert soft-fruit grower; hot chilli dishes because their new boyfriend is Mexican; pepper on virtually everything; curries every Friday because a new curry restaurant has opened nearby.

Many people have food allergies which can manifest as urinary trouble – barley, oats, cereals, white flour, white sugar, bran, fruit, nuts, food colourings, shellfish – the list is endless. There are plenty of good books on allergy, and it's a most interesting subject.

Clothing

The female perineum has an open architecture which is not accidental. Birth needs space, as does intercourse. The vagina retains its health when unimpeded by tight materials and man-made fabrics. Women in past centuries right up to the 1960s were, vaginally speaking, healthy except for the horrors and infections of childbirth, but from then on a decline of daily vaginal health set in. Large companies manufacturing medicines, clothing and underwear have grown fat and profitable on our gullibility, sexual titillation and subsequent poor sexual health.

DON'T WEAR NYLON UNDIES
DON'T WEAR JEANS
DON'T WEAR TIGHTS
DO ALLOW AIR TO YOUR PERINEUM

CHAPTER FOUR

Vaginal Thrush (Monilia)

This is an irritative, milky-looking discharge with curd-like threads, which can wreck your sex life and cause tremendous discomfort. I teach prevention and awareness of the conditions which give rise to thrush. Again, as with all the sections in this chapter, read my other books for full information but abide herein, without questioning, by these rules:

1   DON'T wear tight clothing or nylon underwear.
2   DON'T sit in hot baths.
3   DON'T swim regularly in chlorinated water. Always shower and change into a cool cotton dress/skirt.
4   DON'T drink alcohol if you're very prone to thrush.
5   DON'T eat chocolates or sweets. Cut out sugar.
6   DON'T take any antibiotics for any illness unless you run a preventive course of antifungal pessaries at the same time.
7   DON'T get hot and sweaty, e.g. playing tennis, sunbathing, etc.
8   DON'T sit all day on the edge of office chairs. Sit back and let the vaginal orifice breathe.
9   DON'T remain on the contraceptive pill if thrush has co-incided with it.

All nine points are reasoned on thrush liking warmth, moisture, darkness and sugar, viz:

Q   What is a bath?
A   Hot and wet.
Q   What is in alcohol?
A   Sugar and yeast.
Q   Why can antibiotics cause thrush?

A Because they are not selective in removing bacteria, fungal invasion is more readily achieved.

It pays to have a cervical clearance swab after medical treatment. It pays to practise prevention very rigorously, and in some cases it might pay to take a good long course of Nystatin oral tablets. You will find that some British doctors won't like this, but many American allergy specialists recognize candida (thrush) as an all-over body allergy and prescribe Nystatin without the reservations of the average British general practitioner. You may have to be wily this side of the Atlantic!

In fact, knowing how to make use of the medical profession has become an essential part of lay life. If one doctor can't help you, go to another. This is, of course, easier said than done – except in a health centre, where you can visit any one on duty. Additionally, approach a good private doctor whom one or more friends have recommended. Instead of, or as well as, membership of a private health insurance company, you could arrange with your bank manager to organize a standing order into a separate deposit account for the family's health needs. In this society there are many ways to ensure that you are not entirely dependent upon one doctor or on the National Health Service. The NHS ought to be grateful because more space is left for the truly poorest among us. Contrary to some fashionable beliefs, I believe that going private can be interpreted as a Christian act – going without, yet still paying the National Insurance contributions, which by law we all must.

AMI is an International Health Care Company currently running several large private hospitals in the UK. They now have a system of repayment after treatment in any one of their hospitals tailored over two years to suit the patient's purse. Details can be had by asking for the Director of Finance on 01-486 1266.

I think it is high time that hire purchase terms were brought into use by both hospitals and doctors.

PART TWO
VICTIMS

Introduction

I began counselling in 1978. It was a very natural progression from writing advice and giving advice on the telephone, both of which are self-limiting. Because of the complexities of each woman and the way in which I work, it is impossible to see more than three women a day. Some travel great distances to see me, and others are not fully investigated by the end of the one-hour session, so I always allow plenty of time in between each patient for the vagaries of trains and traffic. Recently one complicated case went on to a two-hour session and this wasn't superfluous chattering. A great deal of questioning, answering, sifting and thinking goes on.

I never ever examine a patient; I am not medically trained. If I feel that previous medical examinations and investigations have not been sufficiently rigorous, then I will refer to an appropriate specialist. To my credit, every patient whom I have referred to any specific specialist has been found to be in medical need. This only goes to show that there are doctors and doctors! It spells out the need for second and third opinions and it spells out the need for an independent assessment. That is how I like to regard myself – an independent assessor. My mind is open for every patient to create her own set of symptoms and problems.

During the hour she will reach into well-researched pockets of my knowledge, but often my list of suggestions at the end will contain a variety of ideas quite beyond the limitations which dominate conventional medicine. I won't categorically rule out anything, except, of course, anything harmful.

It can be helpful to know that the patient is able to meet a bill for, at least, one private specialist consultation and, hopefully, for any investigations. It would also be very helpful if private doctors weren't so damned expensive. The few whom I use charge no more than the appalling London rates that everyone else does, but at least I can trust mine to be honest and expert. It's very hard, I know, to have to accept that you must pay up if you are incapacitatingly ill, but until every doctor within the NHS does a *proper* job – and it's not a matter of resources, it's a matter of time and the doctor's skill – then I do feel that I can only safely recommend such desperate women to trusted specialists. It's that or nothing.

The more private hospitals that are built – just as with videos, televisions etc. – the lower will be the prices. It's a market situation.

I probably send one in five patients to one of the handful of specialists in whom I have total trust. I use a urologist (very rarely), a proctologist (for bowels), an allergist and two gynaecologists. One gynaecologist specializes in super-careful examination and surgery, the other works mostly in the field of hormone replacement therapy. I have once used an acupuncturist and occasionally an excellent private general practitioner, whose surgery facilities are as good as any small hospital. I never use a psychiatrist.

The majority of women who come have already had many X-rays and investigations which have proved negative. This usually means that their own life-style is not suiting their system in some way, e.g. their job, their husband's job, their bathroom routines, etc. Too many women come bearing the results of medical mismanagement and over-prescribing.

Often, the patient has been referred to me by her own doctor. This is always a treat because I know that there is full medical back-up and interest, and a broader medical mind than is the luck of most patients!

I would not think of my approach as being consistent with holistic medicine or naturopathy. The investigation of cystitis does have boundaries of enquiry, but other symptoms in a given patient, say, with sexual bruising – like being underweight – would be likely to have a diet needing investigation.

Listening, thinking, not classifying the patient, are the tools with which I work.

Having been through the mill myself, I am all sympathy, even if at times I express it abruptly in trying to make a patient understand the importance of some point. I, too, would not believe early in my own suffering. I, too, have cut corners and suffered for it.

Many is the patient who thinks that she is 'doing everything, washing as you say, Mrs Kilmartin,' but who on very close questioning just isn't!

I get annoyed with doctors who will keep on investigating in one area, especially American doctors who use urethral dilatation not just once, as if that isn't bad enough, but time after time. Dilatation is still used fashionably, but it should really only be used in a condition called interstitial cystitis. (And don't accept that you have this condition from only one doctor – if two others say that you have it, then you can believe it.)

I get annoyed with patients who accept courses of antibiotics ad nauseam and don't push on any further for constructive help. There is plenty of help available now; there wasn't in 1966!

My home in London has a comfortable room and relaxed atmosphere far removed from the constraints of the usual doctor/patient formalities. Things are said to me that are absolutely impossible in a surgery/desk confrontation. I don't even work off a table. The patient and I face one another over some kind of liquid refreshment from armchairs. My 'suggestion' sheet with its carbon copy paper is usually perched on a pulled up dining chair, and my investigative notes are made on my lap. The room is neat and tidy and very sunny. All patients are greeted by me personally and I put them straight at ease. Accompanying people, mostly husbands, are welcomed and asked whether they would like to sit elsewhere in the house or come in, too. Usually this has been discussed between them prior to arrival and I am always happy to abide by their decision.

Mothers and daughters usually choose to separate, accompanying friends may choose either and husbands always sit in. If there appears any feeling of doubt, I stress the nature of the probingly intimate questions.

The use of the family bathroom is offered immediately. Many patients have had long journeys and may also be thirsty, so whilst they are upstairs I go down and prepare whatever they have requested. The bathroom is a focal point of cleanliness in my house. Even my young son has from an early age been taught, and followed up on, his own hygiene as well as to 'leave the bathroom as he has found it'. He has, from eight years old, taken his turn in the holidays to clean the lavatory, basin and bath. I check his system, too! No one is allowed to antisepticize the lavatory seat or the bath. Every item is carefully wiped free of all cleansing fluid until I am quite satisfied that there can be no perineal contamination by chemicals.

Before patients and in between patients, I clean the lavatory myself. My bathroom is cheerful, with its red-and-white French nursery-rhyme wallpaper and red taps. It's warm and bright and evokes a delight from visitors, and this has a helping hand in continuing the ice-breaking, which started the moment that the hall door was opened.

The objectives of counselling are:

1 To stop the problem/s if possible for all time.
2 To refer to someone who will greatly facilitate this, if found necessary.
3 To stabilize the condition and not allow it to worsen.
4 To improve the daily life quality.
5 To improve upon the existing problem/s.

Compare that with the medical objectives at GP level:

1 Treat this one episode.
2 See if there is anything wrong with the kidneys.

Compare that with the urological objectives:

1 Take an IVP. If negative, refer back to GP.
2 Investigate by cystoscopy. If negative, refer back to GP.
3 If problems continue, suggest dilatation and tranquillizers.

In other words, categorize the patient, and if she blasted well doesn't fit one of the categories – too bad!

Now it would be unfair of me not to acknowledge that there are, thank God, doctors who do try to the utmost of their abilities and who will help the patient search in any way likely to be fruitful. So, if you are a doctor and reading this, then you will know which sort you are, and if you're the latter sort – bravo and thank you!

I'm no feminist or radical; I wear make-up, dresses, high heels and bras. I am just intensely practical. Sick women mean unhappy marriages, strained families, monetary loss and the millions of things likely to go wrong in a household if she can't see to them. Sick women mean many medical hours, drug bills, and are an incessant financial drain on the country.

I must say that I'm the opposite kind of woman from those in past generations. I try very hard to put myself first and not last. (It doesn't always come out quite like that!) If I go under, my family suffers, timetables aren't met, good meals not cooked, etc. I am important;

so is every woman. I think that I must have got this over to my daughter because she recently put a sticker in the car – 'I used to be conceited, but now I'm perfect!'

I digress.

Nevertheless, I'm not so conceited about female health as the new radical local lady doctor, who refused to give me antibiotics for one of my usual awful bouts of sinusitis, and recommended inhaling, then said triumphantly, 'Now what *else* is wrong?'

'Nothing that a *good* doctor wouldn't put right,' I retorted and stalked with tears in my eyes to the door. Next surgery, I went to another branch of the same practice and saw a sympathetic doctor.

Thus I chat, and by the time the patient has settled in her armchair with her drink, she's warmed up and forthcoming. It all takes three or four minutes – no time – and we commence.

Working under paragraph headings is the logical way of eliciting information. According to what the patient says, so I will, after some time, use new headings or discard unnecessary ones. For instance, an unmarried woman of sixty will be less likely (I only say *less* likely) to be having a steady sex life; a newly married girl will not have any injuries from childbirth, although I always ask whether any pregnancy has occurred and been terminated.

All patients have the major headings, as you will see. Everyone starts with 'symptoms'. Until I know exactly what they are sitting in my room complaining about, I can't possibly help. So on this first heading we take time and details. I also leave a space for anything remembered later on.

For the purpose of this book I have enlarged upon my comments so that you can understand how I give my thoughts free range. For instance, I will describe the patient and her background to set each one in the mind, and to outline the highly relevant individual life-style, which does have so much influence. From another viewpoint, you must also understand that I am not doing verbatim reporting off tapes, so the conversations are not described word for word.

Here then, in the rest of the book are some of the secret victims – your friends and relations – of cystitis and thrush. Their names have been changed to preserve anonymity. These are the women whom I forbid and discourage from meeting and chatting over their problems for fear that one will influence the other for the worse.

You will clearly see why: each women is so different from the others. You will also see clearly why cystitis is beyond the doctor's capabilities and limitations of time and insight. If any doctor would be interested, I would come to his area and counsel his persistent cases.

CHAPTER ONE

Miss Mary Smith

The day after Mary Smith telephoned me, I managed to fit her in for a quick appointment. On the phone she had been snuffly and tearful, quite obviously worried and fed up. At twenty-four, she has a job in the City of London with British Telecom as a specialized typist doing work on word processors and other new equipment. Not being too far away from my office, she arrived promptly at 3 p.m. the next day and was a little more chirpy, and pleased to be coming to talk over her problem.

Very much a young girl, she lives her spare time in accordance with her boyfriend Kevin's life-style. He is an unemployed credit controller filling in his days with bar work. Kevin and Mary have been together for five years and have a double bed in her room at the flat which her mother rents from an inner-London council. Kevin sleeps with her there most nights. He plays football in the winter and cricket in the summer, so that social life for both of them in the evenings is usually in the bar of a social sports club or a public house.

Mary's mother doesn't work and obviously succeeds in making a comfortable home, to which Kevin and Mary happily return. Mary is quite short, probably under five feet, and she wore a midnight blue silky polyester office dress with boots. Removing her warm winter coat, she sat on the edge of the armchair without relaxing back at all.

Symptoms

Thrush, with the creamy, irritative discharge. She rang me because the initial three-day course of Canesten pessaries had stung and hadn't worked. The GP had prescribed a further, lengthier course and today, the second day, was at last showing results. She felt less depressed because the vagina had stopped stinging. The GP hadn't examined her but had taken her word that it was thrush, from what she remembered of her only previous attack eight years ago aged sixteen.

She also got bouts of burning urine with frequency. Sometimes there is a dragging pain but she has never bled with it. These bouts occurred roughly between the ages of seventeen and twenty-three. All urine tests are negative.

Urological history

MSUs – all negative.
No other investigations.

Gynaecological history

Periods normal.
No operations.

Pregnancies and babies

1 pregnancy – miscarried in 1980.
1st coil fitted in 1980.
2nd coil fitted in 1983.

Sex

4/5 times a week and has no side effects unless coupled with a high alcohol intake.
Mary wears sanitary towels not Tampax.
She bathes twice a week and has stand-up basin washes in between.

Clothing

She wears tights but has all-cotton underwear. Trousers are worn occasionally but she never wears jeans.

Diet and liquid intake

Diet is not good, reference thrush, and the alcohol intake is very high. With bars featuring as the dominant entertainment, Mary drinks *3½ pints* of lager plus Bacardi and Coke most nights. She can also be persuaded to follow these with shorts. If she's not drinking alcohol, she's drinking Coke, lemonade or orange juice – all canned and sweetened.

Mary does have a sweet tooth and will happily demolish sweets, chocolates and gateaux.

Hygiene

This isn't good but then, since she has no bladder infections, I can't wag my finger too hard. Mary doesn't wash at all after passing a stool but recently she has begun to attempt some hygiene after sex. This is decidedly more sporadic than the sex!

General health

Being an epileptic, Mary is permanently on control drugs. Fits this year have been totally absent, which I understand is a record, and is attributed hopefully to the drugs.

Job

Although she says that she walks around in the office, she spends most of the day on her hard typist's chair with its small back-rest. The office is very warm in winter from the modern central heating.

My suggestions

1. The string of the coil has been known to encourage and harbour bacteria. Watch out for this hazard in the future.
2. Thrush breeds in warmth and moisture. It loves to eat sugar.
3. The opposite of warm and moist is cool and dry. Aim to keep the perineum cool and dry.
4. Tights cause retention of moisture from any perineal sweating. Wear stockings and suspenders – they can be very pretty these days.
5. Whenever you have thrush don't get in the bath at all. A bath is hot and wet and encourages inflammation. Your stand-up washes are best.
6. At home, curl up in your armchair without pants. Wear a long cosy skirt and try to sit with the legs apart and the skirt hiding all!
7. Thrush loves sugar. Cut out sweets, chocolates and gateaux.

8   For the same reason, cut out canned drinks and sweetened juices.

9   The same goes for alcohol. Alcohol converts to sugar. Cut out alcohol.

10 Keep your water intake high, especially on hot beaches and in hot offices. Dehydration causes over acid urine which burns but has no bacteria.

11 After passing a stool and after intercourse, wash as I demonstrated.

12 Cut pubic hair to ½ inch with scissors to help the perineum stay dry.

13 Hard chairs frequently used remove air access to the perineum.

14 They 'squash' the perineal skin and can make it swollen.

15 Sit back in chairs, keep thighs apart and let air circulate.

16 I feel that the negative bouts of urinary discomfort are being triggered by too much alcohol, coupled with sex.

17 Thrush can 'ping-pong' between sexual partners. If attacks begin to occur regularly despite all this other help, then Kevin should get tested.

18 Watch out for bedclothes heat, e.g. Terylene duvets, nylon nighties and sheets. Stick to cotton and sleep naked next to Kevin.

19 Use VD units for thrush examinations. Just say that you think you have a discharge.

My comments

Despite a simple enough history-taking session, I feel it worthwhile in a young woman to point out a number of possible health hazards for future reference. For instance, Mary does now sleep in blankets and a short cotton nightie, but she might decide one day to change so I forewarned.

Someone older in her office had already discussed the high alcohol intake and had suggested Perrier, so here I was seconding the good advice. I'm not advocating utter abstention for ever but for a thrush victim the amount of sugar ingested is very important and should be kept at a reasonable or low level.

Modern office seating and routines can quite definitely be added to the hazards of today's life-style. Office typing means sitting for long periods of time on hard acrylic-fibre chairs. The man-made fibres give no chance for the skin to breathe and, added to the hardness of the chair continuously squashing the perineum, it is a daily thrush trigger.

Alcohol and sex are time-honoured causes of cystitis/urinary discomfort. Alcohol is a diuretic which encourages the renal organs to make and expel urine. If you don't replace the expelled body liquid with glasses of water you will start to pass short amounts of strong, coloured, acid urine. Sexual activity will rub the acidized urethra and bladder, irritating both of them still further. No antibiotics are needed, nor will they help; only large amounts of water. Water will deflame the skin and dilute the urine.

Mary is not yet a real 'victim' – she's a pre-victim. Hopefully this very common case history will alert many millions of girls and young women to caring for and about their health instead of capitulating to boyfriends, social pressures and life-style hazards. Mary's early and sporadic bouts of discomfort will now be averted and permanent trouble avoided.

CHAPTER TWO

Mrs Peggy Watson and Derek

Mrs Watson's vivacity far outshone her fifty-eight years. She positively sparkled with life, and her blonde hair and cheerful make-up were matched in a polka-dot red-on-white summer dress and high heels. Chatty and outgoing, looking me straight in the eye as though she met me every day, she explained how her long journey had gone and requested only a glass of water – apparently she drinks a lot of it.

Derek, sixty years old, her husband for thirty-seven years, is going to take an early retirement next week from college lecturing in management studies. Peggy says that she will have no trouble in keeping him busy!

Three days a week from 10–4, Peggy thoroughly enjoys her rep work for Phillips Electrical in a south coast store. She has a good lunch-break and can sit down whenever she feels tired. Very luckily, her son works in the travel agency business, and this enables her to take fairly sensational holidays – sometimes without Derek, who stays behind to look after the cat. Last year it was America, this year Peggy went to Australia, Hong Kong, Thailand and heaven knows where else, meeting relatives en route.

Hobbies are simple: reading, housework and, when there were no health troubles, she used to swim in the sea creek at the bottom of her garden.

All in all it was difficult to see why she needed counselling, for here was a very attractive and lively lady.

Symptoms

Thirty-six years of cystitis, painful and frequent but no bleeding. Attacks averaged three to four a year, except in her two pregnancies and the first year on the Pill. Cystitis began 6 months after marriage. Although every attack makes her shivery, she has only just had her first temperature. She has never had thrush that she knows of and has never been checked for it. Before the menopause in 1978–9 she was prone to headaches, but since 1979 has been free of them. She felt that they were related to the Pill. Doctors think that she has a 'sensitive bladder'.

Peggy bought my first book 12 years ago and the latest book only last week.

On returning from her month away travelling she commenced an attack of cystitis after three days, and although it was treated with antibiotics and self-help, she is still 'twingeing' three months later. This is her reason for visiting me and requesting counselling. She wants ideas on this attack and its aftermath, and also any light we can throw on why she has had a 36-year history of cystitis.

Urological history

Mid-stream urine specimens: Lots. Some negative. Some positive E.Coli.
Intravenous pyleogram: One. 12 years ago. Negative.
Cystoscopy: One. 12 years ago. Negative.
No Dilatations.

Gynaecological history

Her periods began at 11 years old and came every two weeks or whenever she was in motion, e.g. on a bus or playing sport. She was treated with hormones at this early age and had no further trouble. Menopause took only a year, without a single hot flush to boast of and no difficult moments. Peggy, even now, can't believe how very fortunate she was, neither, I suspect, can we. She has never had a D&C.

Babies and pregnancies

One boy, 1950. No labour pains, no stitches, easy birth but six weeks later, needed cauterization because of an infection in the uterus. This cleared.
One boy, 1955. Birth took ten minutes and she was fully dressed

when it happened. No labour pains at all and no stitches or tears. The hospital accounted for her undoubted abilities in childbirth by crediting her with a perfectly round pelvic cavity.

Contraceptives

Over the years has used Rendalls Pessaries, the sheath and the Pill. Peggy was on the Pill for ten years.

Sex

Very enjoyable, lasting up to an hour two or three times a week all her marriage, except during attacks, and would still be doing so if the current attack had cleared properly. For 12 years, since reading my first book she has used KY Jelly.

(At this point, I am going to revert to the exact order of events in the counselling session.)

Liquid intake

Drinks lots of water. In between attacks Peggy enjoys a glass of dry sherry each night before dinner but hasn't had one for the last three months.

Clothing

Conventional and good – no tights or jeans. She wears cotton underwear and travelled by train and taxi without any pants! (Bit risky this, I thought, and told her so.)

General health and habits

Good. Peggy has always had loose bowels, and two or three times a day extra to the main motion there are likely to be smaller bowel movements, usually whilst passing water. She can't remember a time when this has not happened. Her appendix has been removed and there is no diabetes.

Until my book arrived last Saturday (it has been most intelligently read), she only washed after the major motion each day, *not the two or three smaller ones*. Her daily washing process until last Saturday was as follows:

Using baby soap and hands only, no cloths or cotton wool, she has always stood over a towel soaping and splashing the entire perineum – no cloths, no spraying, just splashing hands. The towel on the floor is not used for drying; she gets another one. She baths each morning and at no other time.

This current attack and events leading to it

Peggy arrived back from her month's Australasian holiday on a Monday lunchtime in March.

On getting inside the front door:

1 She washed as described above and had a short sleep.
2 Later that night she bathed, went to bed, had a short session of intercourse.
3 Wednesday night – a lengthier sex session, 45–60 minutes.
4 Thursday morning at 8 a.m., cystitis. She immediately began a course of antibiotics, which were already in the house, and then waited two weeks before going for an MSU because the attack did not fully go. The MSU showed E.Coli.

In all, between March and June, three urine samples were taken. The first two showed E.Coli, the third was negative and, antibiotics were therefore only stopped after the third sample.

During this time, early April to late June, she bought and used medicated baby wipes and ate pounds of strawberries from the local pick-em-yourself nurseries.

We don't know, because a urine sample was not taken, whether there was E.Coli or simply excessive uric acid, with the sexual trigger bearing responsibility for the 8 a.m. cystitis on that Thursday morning. It may have been all three. Peggy says that she bathed directly before last week's clear urine sample but would not have done so directly before taking the first two, so we might argue that E.Coli was not actually up in the bladder urine. Perhaps E.Coli was transferred into the samples straight off her perineal (outside) skin as the urine flowed outwards and over this faecally contaminated area.

The constantly aggravating twingeing could be over-acid urine from the strawberries, skin reaction to medicated baby wipes and/ or soap-aggravated reaction from her poor washing procedure.

As we went downstairs discussing the strawberries and the amount she had eaten, I remembered that I had not taken a food and liquid intake section.

Food intake

Eats very little red meat, but lots of turkey and chicken, THREE eggs a day and lots of soft fruit. If Peggy goes on a high-protein diet, her diarrhoea becomes acute.

My suggestions

1 Having just taken three months' worth of antibiotics, a thrush check would be in order.
2 Have a full vaginal check.
3 Ask for a special survey of the state of the vaginal epithelium (skin) in case there is any atrophy (ageing) due to lowering hormone balance following menopause.
4 I gave a gynaecologist's name. He would do all this but, of course, the VD/genito-urinary clinic would test just as well. Hormones, however, aren't up their street unless the condition is so severe that they write a referral within the hospital or a letter to the patient's own GP with her cooperation.
5 If Peggy has another attack, she should take the bicarbonate of soda as instructed in the management sequence because this will help alkalize the urine. It will also help reverse an allergic reaction and remove the conditions of acidity which enable E. Coli to grow. Cymalon will help similarly.
6 Only take underwear off indoors. Air outside, especially in busy city streets, carries lots of bacteria. I certainly wouldn't have come on such a long journey without wearing pants.
7 Only eat soft fruit in small amounts and space your intake. Be ready to counteract and dilute over-acid urine.
8 In view of the sensitive bladder and runny bowels, which are even worse on an all-protein diet, is Peggy allergic to protein?
9 For all this week remove turkey, chicken and eggs from the diet. See whether the bowel movements are reduced each day. Ring me in a week's time to tell me, please.
10 Is Peggy allergic in particular to eggs? Allergic responses to favourite foods are well known.
11 For two months:
   (a) Wash as now instructed not as you used to.
   (b) No chicken, turkey or eggs (reintroduce them in small quantities on a strict rotation-and-gap diet).

(c) No more strawberries this year and a little less wholemeal bread.

12 For this week only take one level teaspoon of bicarbonate in water or jam at night (Peggy has no heart problem). If the twingeing is being caused by acidity or allergic responses, the bicarb will counteract both. Cymalon would also do.

13 Twingeing could also be being caused by thrush after all those antibiotics, and we certainly need to know if low-grade thrush is present.

14 Washing was awful. ANY bowel movement at all needs the full bottle-washing process.

My comments

This took just over an hour and a half. It was complicated but very interesting and I felt like Sherlock Holmes's sister! Have we come to an understanding of Peggy's 36-year history? Have we broken the back of this year's attack?

Peggy has *always* eaten that many eggs, *always* had two or three bowel movements every day, *always* washed that inefficiently.

She says that after every course of antibiotics she has usually felt a little hot and itchy but never bothered with a vaginal check for thrush because eventually it has gone. After three months of antibiotics now, though, she certainly needs a thrush check.

If Peggy follows through my suggestions, there could be a dramatic change in her daily body habits. Her general health is good, so we are not looking for changes here. With my head stuck optimistically out, I foresee those changes happening in just one week. We'll see.

Follow-up – August

Mrs Watson reported the following:
- A visit to the local VD unit, which showed good vaginal health with no sign of thrush or bacteria.
- No soft fruit, eggs, chicken, turkey have been eaten but her bowels have worked as before. Disappointing for me.
- Excellent bottle-washing routines should now prevent further E.Coli bladder infections no matter how many times her bowels move in a day. I am not inclined to pursue the allergy line any further. My interest in any allergies to eggs, chicken etc., ends here in her case.

- Twingeing is still occurring. There is no pattern as, for instance, a definite time of day or night; it occurs irregularly. Liquid intake at home or at work is good and even in warm weather she is certainly not dehydrating.
- A teaspoonful of bicarbonate of soda is taken at night in water.
- Today, Peggy had a very negative five-minute session with an NHS urology registrar who declined to make any suggestions at all about the twingeing.
- Peggy is admitting for the first time to me that she is going through a stressful period. Apparently it is to do with work and it has been so since she returned from Australia. I put it to her that if vaginal atrophy was in its early stages, an inexperienced hormone 'eye' such as that of the doctor in the VD unit might not be specialized enough to spot it. Hormones change by the day and hour and cycle. Peggy's periods stopped in 1978. The slowly diminishing hormone output in her body may only now be showing its first symptom. Lack of hormones can account for urethral symptoms. Although she hadn't actually seen the gynaecologist whom I had previously recommended, I have now changed my mind and have recommended a specialist with a more finely tuned hormone eye. This man is currently conducting some more work into urethral involvement as an indication of hormone malfunction.

   The stress from the job plus the natural menopausal ageing may now be behind the twingeing. She has indicated that she will ring this specialist tomorrow for an early appointment.

Follow-up – September

Peggy made the appointment but severe burning urine that morning prevented her from travelling to London.

Peggy is a first-class counselling patient. She has followed to the letter my suggestions and has also kept her general practitioner fully informed. He, in turn, has become very interested in the progress and suggestions, even instituting the following investigations and suggestions of his own to back up mine:

- He has referred her to a Hampshire allergy clinic, believing, as I do still, that some foods may be disagreeing with her.

- He has done a blood hormone evaluation test and, sure enough, the oestrogen count is lowering, although medically acceptable in a post-menopausal lady of 58.

With urethral symptoms of twingeing and burning, though, those lowered hormone levels can certainly assume responsibility. Peggy is going to receive hormone treatment from the local general practitioner. He may choose a vaginal cream like Dinoestrol, which only has a localized vaginal action or, in view of the blood hormone levels, he may choose some tablet which will influence their levels throughout the body and assist the urethral burning.

I favour the latter. I have known many women in this situation derive great relief from symptoms with a hormone implant, which is a timed release of hormones into the system – lasting about six months then repeated.

Peggy has made good investigative headway and is therefore very confident. She will be in touch again.

Follow-up – mid-November

Peggy has not yet started the hormone treatment because a chance MSU taken by her GP when the twingeing was particularly bad showed heavy E.Coli urinary infection despite her now superb hygiene. Subsequent MSUs have shown a continuous E.Coli, regardless of the large doses of antibiotics now being taken.

What an unexpected turn of events! Peggy, however, is now possessed of an enquiring and persistent mind with her new knowledge of cystitis, born from re-reading my books and seeing me. More chance entered the story last week.

She was in the large staff ladies' cloakroom at the department store where she does three days a week part-time in the electrical department, when a colleague came out of a cubicle and they started chatting.

'I'd be fine,' said the colleague, 'if only I could get rid of this wretched cystitis.'

Peggy said, 'Do you know what is causing it?'

'E.Coli urinary infection,' the colleague replied.

'Snap,' said Peggy.

'Also,' said the colleague, 'I've never ever had cystitis before I came here to work.'

Peggy's mind flashed back to the start of her own period of symptom continuity, not the times of years ago when it was more sporadic. Her E. Coli could also be traced back to the time she started in the store. She returned to the electrical department and asked a few women that afternoon whether they had ever had cystitis. Five employees in that department alone were even now on antibiotics for E.Coli cystitis and often had it!

At this amazing point I rang to do this supposedly final follow-up. Peggy and I decided on a plan of action:

1 First thing Monday she is going to the staff nurse to tell her about it, and I have asked her to ask the nurse to request a full council health department and a full private laboratory water and tap survey of the store, particularly the large staff ladies' cloakroom.

2 Pin up a notice, in a relevant place such as the cloakroom, with Peggy's phone number requesting that any one with E.Coli cystitis phone her at home. This would give a fuller idea of the numbers involved. The notice is to remain up for 2 weeks.

3 Ask the staff nurse to requisition me for a hygiene lecture to the female staff and the toilet cleaners.

Peggy puts paper on the seat when she uses it and she now keeps a bottle at work to wash properly each time she visits the lavatory because of her temperamental bowel movements. I now have no reason to suspect her own hygiene so we must look elsewhere for the source of the bacteria.

Toilet seats, flush handles, taps, towels, hot-air dryer knobs, all can carry trace amounts of faecal material from women whose hand hygiene is poor. Just think of the thousands of women you have seen in public cloakrooms who come out of lavatories and turn on the taps only to pass their hands through the running tap water, turn it off and dry their hands on filthy towels or by pressing the hot air knob! In a work situation where women are more likely to pass a stool there than at home, such a cloakroom is likely to have more faecal bacteria than an average shoppers' cloakroom. Most women shoppers 'hang on' until they are home before allowing a bowel movement.

Peggy has a lifelong sensitivity to attacks of cystitis but now the pace is increasing and currently continuous. True, her hormone levels are lowering and her skin will not throw off bacterial invasion so well, but other factors like the situation amongst other staff and her now expert bowel hygiene cause a rapid re-think of the situation. Investigators of cystitis MUST be flexible; this book has to show that. The investigations of the cloakrooms and the number of victims in the store staff are of riveting interest.

Follow-up – late November

Peggy spoke to the nurse, who promised to speak to Personnel and put up the notices. After two weeks nothing had transpired – no notices, no contact from the nurse and no notification of any tap survey. A colleague says that the staff cloakroom is only cleaned twice a week and Peggy says that it is usually dirty.

She has given in her notice and leaves shortly. I was going to suggest this soon but she has already seen to it. Also next week she has an appointment with a microbiologist with a special interest in urinary bacterial infections. Peggy has been solidly on Negram since September but is still twingeing if not actually having to do the full management of an attack procedure.

Her bowels are obviously highly sensitive. Perhaps the membrane is raw enough to be allowing E.Coli infiltration of the kidneys and bladder via the bloodstream. Perhaps not. Perhaps there is a small diverticulum (extra pouch on the bladder) which is harbouring E.Coli. Perhaps just leaving the department store and its dirty staff lavatories will stop the continuous E.Coli bladder infections.

I still pursued the idea of hormone treatment. The lowered hormone levels will predispose her to less healthy skin, which will harbour bacteria. Topping up these levels would only enhance other work suggested by the microbiologist.

It is twelve years since Peggy last had an IVP or cystoscopy. Another set of investigations now would be of interest.

Follow-up – mid-January

Peggy saw Dr Missell, the microbiologist, at the end of November. The doctor listened and talked but did not instigate any further tests except another urine culture. This was negative, the first to be so for months. She felt that although I may yet be right about a diverticulum, for the time being she wanted Peggy to pass urine every 2½ hours without fail in case the bladder was not emptying itself completely each time. This action would prevent any remaining urine from harbouring bacteria. Peggy did not tell her about the dirty staff lavatories at work, since she was leaving on 1 December anyway.

As a result of the clean urine culture, Dr Missell has put Peggy on to one nightly capsule of Macrodantin for a month, which is now up. Peggy is no longer sore and feels very well. She waits in the earnest hope that all is now set for a cystitis-free future! Her hygiene is excellent and she is without the background worry of dirty staff lavatories at work. She devoutly follows the frequent urination suggestion.

She has said that it was marvellous to talk every step through with me, especially the hygiene and the work situation. Hormonally nothing has been done because it finally proved unnecessary but it should always be kept as a reserve thought at Peggy's age.

That her worst years of cystitis began when she started work at the store and stopped when she stopped working there is tremendously coincidental. Even my hygiene procedure didn't work for her in the three months following our September consultation. It was that fact that made me wonder whether she would benefit by leaving work. Our consultation also sparked her off thinking about the staff lavatories and, together with that wonderful chance meeting with her colleague over the basins, helped cement her idea to give in notice.

As with so many cystitis victims there is seldom one solitary cause for their cystitis. In Peggy's case it may have been three:

1   Poor perineal hygiene
1   Ineffectual bladder emptying
3   E.Coli external contamination from dirty lavatories.

Peggy and Derek are having plenty of intercourse and obviously loving it. Life is as good as it was in the heady days of 1948!

CHAPTER THREE

Mrs Florence Southam

Arriving 15 minutes ahead of time, just right really, Mrs Southam was concise in explaining a train hold-up, which she had resolved by leaping off into the taxi queue ahead of less decisive fellow passengers. She looked every inch the professional, dedicated, life-long business woman. Her lovely lightweight wool suit matched her image and her colouring. Dark high heels set off the eau-de-nil suit, and a practical, tidy hair-style framed a lively face with blonde hair.

She chatted with an assured gusto and happily drank two cups of coffee. She didn't need the bathroom and sat elegantly in my armchair, a picture of good health. Married to Roger for the last 7 years, she is now 55 and has worked for a major multinational computer company since 1949. Her work within the company has naturally varied over the years but she has now been in the computer room for some time. This room has a carefully controlled atmosphere so that the sensitive computers, processors and terminals are not influenced by voltage changes from the grid system or by humidity. The room is therefore dry and the temperature on the cool side.

Roger has also worked all his life in this company, so they have a great mutual enjoyment; one could almost describe the work as their baby – they don't have any children. Roger is a Fulham football supporter and now sits in the very same seat in the stadium as his father before him. Florence goes sometimes, but her great interest outside work is horse-racing. Living in Richmond, just outside London, she is well placed for Saturday racing at several racecourses and she places bets both at weekends and during the week.

A high IQ means that she loves being not just busy but also involved in the figurework of big business, and involved in the intricacies of betting and form which mark the true punter.

Retirement, therefore, due in five weeks' time, might pose a problem. This woman has gone out to work every week of her adult life – there have been no weeks off to have babies, care for old folk or simply take a lengthy break. I wondered how she was going to fill in her days to match her active brain and body. She quickly began a list of activities and obviously has the whole thing planned and under control; whoever or whatever receives her time and energy is going to be very lucky.

Symptoms

Burning skin along the perineum; she doesn't feel that the urine is burning. The skin is tender and dry and has been worsening in fits and starts since 1982. Weekdays used to be symptom-free, with weekends providing the worst time, but since February, that pattern has ended. There has been an additional cyclical pattern to it since the hysterectomy in July 1981. In the last 6 years Florence has had 2 full-blown attacks of cystitis. She has no headaches, no joint or limb pains and no thrush.

The week prior to seeing me on a Monday had been difficult, with burning and twingeing, but on Saturday she had taken six Aspro and drunk a stack of water, and by the next day all discomfort had gone. She was completely comfortable for our counselling.

Urological history

Very limited. Mid-stream urine specimens have only been taken 3 times and were completely clear. No IVP has been done and no cystoscopy performed.

Florence has seen one London urologist who, at private consultation, thought that a polyp in the bladder might be the answer but wanted her under an anaesthetic for purposes of investigative cystoscopy. She was booked into a private clinic the day before the operation so that an anaesthetist could visit and discuss whether the 25mg Tofranil tablets which ease her occasional bouts of agoraphobic behaviour should be taken the night before an anaesthetic. She duly arrived at lunchtime and booked in. By 5 p.m., when the consultant anaesthetist had failed to turn up, she enquired of the sister when he might be expected. Sister replied that he wasn't coming anyway, he was on holiday!

Florence's indignation at what she considered deception by the urologist and the extra night's clinic expenses were enough to make her check out of the clinic and take herself off the urologist's operation list. She has not seen a urologist since then. In any case, she remains certain that she has a good strong bladder.

Gynaecological history

Periods began aged 13 and were heavy right up to the hysterectomy. In 1978 she entered hospital for a D&C, and the gynaecologist told her afterwards that he had decided not to remove some fibroids which he had found because they would be quite likely to shrink in time. He was right to some degree, but after the menopause, which took place between 1978 and 1980, another gynaecologist thought that they had not shrunk enough and because Florence's stomach was distended he recommended a hysterectomy. This was done in 1981.

Following the hysterectomy, the GP has tried Orthodinoestrol vaginal hormone creams and Prempack C hormone tablets, but Florence remains a slightly awkward patient when it comes to tablets and medications (she hates taking them) and didn't think that the cream had helped anyway, so the GP's efforts went unrewarded.

Self-help

It may prove to be largely inapplicable since cystitis and burning has only followed the hysterectomy. She has no discharges nor was there any history of urological or gynaecological disorders prior to this period of time.

Diet

This turned out to reveal some interest. Coinciding roughly with the hysterectomy was the closure of the small café oppose the office where Florence always went for lunch and, hating the thought of going into the staff canteen each day, she began to take her own sandwiches. From her youth, Florence had been hooked on banana sandwiches because that was her mother's favourite – no other sort was ever made! Florence's fruit intake each day is:

    a grapefruit for breakfast

    1½ bananas in the sandwiches

1 apple
a bowl of stewed fruit and cream or custard every night for dessert
1 orange eaten before going up to bed

She enjoys two or three sweet sherries before dinner each evening.
Florence eats a lot of chocolate, something like two bars a week and
a half pound on Saturdays. She uses salt and pepper on every
mouthful of food at all meals and, up until trouble began in the early
1980s, she would down about 14 cups of tea a day. This has been
cut down to about six a day plus two coffees. Amazingly, Florence
had not counted frequency amongst her symptoms. She must have
a very strong bladder! At weekends she'll drink more sherries and
have wine on Saturday night and at Sunday lunch.

Florence's 83-year-old mother was a great banana fan, also had
a hysterectomy, but had lots of cystitis and is severely crippled with
arthritis.

Sex

Doesn't appear to be having any adverse effect at all and is regularly
enjoyed whenever symptoms wane a little. A lubricant is used to
help with the dryness, and the two or three sessions a week usually
last 10 or 15 minutes. Symptoms do not return following intercourse
and this may be because of the KY Jelly and the shortness of
intercourse.

General health

Is good and Florence is seldom, if ever, off sick. She prefers being
very busy, but following a close family death some time ago takes a
Tofranil anti-depressant tablet at night. Two weeks ago she set out
to go shopping at Harrods and reached the front door, only to
become fearful of the crush of people enclosed in the building
entrance and so she had to come away very quickly.

Hygiene

Obviously fine since there are no discharges and no urinary infections ever reported. Florence has always soaped her entire perineum
with Knight's Castile soap, and I warned her off using it in the front
part of the perineum now that her skin was burning and probably
less tolerant than before the hysterectomy. She had lent my book to

a friend some time ago and it hasn't been returned, so she bought another one from me to re-read.

My suggestions

Very few:

- Check for hormone deficiency following hysterectomy and menopause.
- Ageing skin does not tolerate excess acidity such as that produced by Florence's daily fruit intake.
- I gave the name of a hormone specialist for further work here, but Florence is reluctant and would rather try to rearrange her diet first.
- Hygiene was good enough but it's better to drop the soaping of the entire perineum now, only soap the back passage.
- Cut out the fruit and alcohol for two weeks and then slowly reintroduce them little by little.

My comments

This was a twofold result. On the one hand, the hysterectomy date matching the start of symptoms clearly showed a hormonal relationship to the burning; and on the other, the extra daily bananas in Florence's sandwiches following the café's closure might have been the final straw on a heavily fruit-laden, acidized urinary system. Florence had mentioned the fruit to her GP but he had passed it over as being insignificant.

If the combination of ageing skin and over-acidity are causing the trouble, we shall only know which one it is when Florence has removed the fruit and alcohol for two weeks. It may do the trick, but if not then the hormone levels must be investigated and if necessary treated with due deference to Florence's dislike of medications!

Follow-up – October

Florence rang back to say very simply that whilst she appreciated that future hormone treatment may prove necessary, it wasn't now. Having revised the fruit and alcohol intake and brought it down to a lower amount, all her twinges and soreness have stopped completely. Her GP stands in some disbelief at the stoppage of symptoms following the dietary revision but accepts that the proof of the pudding is in the eating. Fair enough! Florence is well now and that's all that matters. YOUR comfort is the only acceptable yardstick for YOU, not anyone else.

CHAPTER FOUR

Miss Chrissie Peatbridge and Don

Chrissie Peatbridge, aged 23 and unmarried, is a journalist writing feature articles for friendly magazine editors in London. For the past year, her boyfriend Don, a television director aged 33, has not lived with her but for the three years prior to that, he had.

Chrissie came partly to interview me for an article on thrush and partly for me to counsel her, since she is also a thrush victim. She has short, straight fair hair and a classic Grecian face with pretty profile, and she had dressed top to toe in white – blouse, skirt, stockings and ribbon-tied flat pumps. Looking every inch a dancer, which indeed turned out to be her major hobby – she has almost made it a second career except that she doesn't earn her living at it. Three evenings a week are devoted to contemporary dance; another evening is spent on her new interest, Tsai Chi, a form of self-defence by martial arts; and on spare nights she goes to the theatre, mainly to see dance companies currently in town. Being a journalist fosters an interest in books, so she reads on trains and in between events.

Don is also into modern dance as an active participant but one would not find this unusual since his directing specialty is for dance and music programmes. Don also has thrush.

Symptoms

Classic thrush: hot curdy discharge, intense irritation, which makes her scratch and draw blood. The perineum and pubic hair area (pubis) are all sore and inflamed. She has been like this for the last three years or so with remission periods of about 5–6 weeks between attacks. The increase in attacks seems to have coincided with Don moving in, and although she had a few attacks prior to this, they had been far less frequent. Symptoms, she says, are worse in summer. She also gets occasional bouts of eczema and psoriasis but not too badly. Thrush has been shown on swabs many times and responds well to local medication for the vagina.

Urological history

None – no problems. Chrissie does feel that if she wasn't washing after intercourse and passing urine, she might be a cystitis victim because she does occasionally twinge from bruising after a heavy sex session.

Gynaecological history

Periods began at 13 and were moderately heavy, using up just over one packet of STs. Occasionally there was pain but rarely a problem. She has had plenty of vaginal swabs and reckons to know all the best VD units between Bedford and London – very wise even though she doesn't sleep around. She has had cervical smears and Pill check-ups every few years. She has never had a D&C.

Contraceptives

At 16, she went on the Pill, Eugynon – for its contraceptive value, not for help with periods – but headaches made her change to Microgynon. She tries to have six-month breaks from it every few years and is due now for a break.

In the breaks she has tried the cap and fought and lost a battle with it! Because of her dancing, the muscles in the pelvic region are very strong and the cap has gone walkabout during intercourse, and although she never became pregnant, she reckoned she was lucky! Condoms have also been tried but they brought on 'boyfriend's allergy'! Amazing how many men have a condom allergy these days! It used to be THE method of birth control.

Sex

Is comfortable, enjoyable and happens on average two to three times a week. Intercourse does not stop for thrush.

Babies and pregnancies

None.

General health

Excellent. She is very fit. Eczema and psoriasis are occasional blots.

Food intake

Chrissie is vegetarian but will eat fish. She eats a great deal of fruit, sometimes 2½ pounds a day. She has no sugar in tea or coffee. White bread was stopped some years ago because she felt that it was the reason behind some minor stomach trouble, which has since cleared. Every so often, she eats Mars bars.

Liquid intake

She doesn't drink alcohol, but maybe once a month might have a couple of glasses of wine although she doesn't really enjoy it since it often makes her feel nauseous. Each day Chrissie reckons to drink two cans of Diet Coke but after a dance work-out she usually has Perrier or other mineral water.

Clothes

Chrissie usually wears stockings and suspenders, and her bikini briefs have a cotton gusset on top of the nylon. She sometimes wears baggies and always puts on the bottoms of a track suit after dancing to stop her muscles from going into spasm. Dancing, modern dancing, is always done in lycra leotards because body line is so important. Nothing is worn underneath them. She spends between six and eight hours a week in leotards. She occasionally wears jeans and tights.

Hygiene

A ten-minute bath is taken four times a week. In addition, she showers three nights a week after dancing. Her pubic hair is free-range and never shortened.

Don

Has had thrush diagnosed, and when Chrissie has thrush he can usually tell her she has it because the penis becomes pink and itchy. He also has a very rumbly stomach.

My suggestions

1 With thrush, eczema, psoriasis, stomach trouble from white bread and nausea from wine, maybe some allergy tests in the future might prove interesting, especially food allergy testing. I gave the name of an allergist working in this field.

2 Change bikini briefs for total cotton and remove them to allow air access to the perineum when at home.

3 Don't wear trousers or jeans at all. That tracksuit bottom can be discarded in favour of a long, warm wrap-around skirt that will allow air to the perineum but still keep the dancing muscles warm.

4 Free-range pubic hair harbours warmth and sweat just like fibreglass insulation in the loft. It is also another air barrier. Cut it and keep it to ½ inch with scissors.

5 Baths provide the conditions in which thrush thrives – warmth and moisture. Stop bathing for two months altogether and then only have one bath a week. And give up the bubble-bath, naughty girl!

6 After dancing don't shower. Use the bottle method to cool the perineum and remove the sweat.

7 Leotards are death! For a thrush-prone woman to wear them at all is crazy, never mind six to eight hours a week.

8 Dance in something else. Chrissie replied and explained why this would be very difficult.

9 Diet Coke still contains a sweetener – just drink mineral water. After two months don't adhere so strictly to this suggestion but do make sure still to bear it in mind.

10 Even fruit, especially in that quantity, contains sugar. Cut the fruit down to one piece a day.

11 When thrush is present you MUST NOT have intercourse. There are two reasons why not:
   (a) The rubbing during intercourse causes heat and swelling.
   (b) Thrush is a sexually transmitted disease, as both she and Don realize.

12 Don has never had treatment for his diagnosed thrush. He should ask for Nystatin oral tablets, and he and Chrissie ought to take a course each to run concurrently.

13 The Pill exacerbates thrush. Have a six-month break now, whilst trying to reorganize the life-style.

14 Exercise, excessive exercise, causes bodily and perineal heating. It can encourage thrush to spread along the perineum and down the inside thigh.

15 Try: after dancing, remove leotard, wash by the cool water-bottle process, put on a long skirt, leave pants off, then there shouldn't be any need to shower, especially after a stand-up wash.

My comments

Despite having had occasional bouts of thrush before meeting and living with Don, the situation is now far from bearable and must be brought under control. Simple changes like point 15 will help bring this about by swinging away from Chrissie's previous routines after dancing. She would sit around in the tracksuit bottoms, keeping warm for the sake of the muscles, showering finally and putting on underwear. This all helps to maintain the ideal conditions for thrush of warmth and moisture.

A lot of intercourse, as she would have had following the start of her relationship with Don three years ago, causes much vaginal/perineal heat and inflammation, encouraging the almost continual breeding of thrush. Without condoms to restrain Chrissie's fungus to her body, Don's bodily contact with hers would have enabled easy transference of bacteria, and this has happened.

The combination of the sex and the dancing are, in my opinion, most likely of all to be the root causes of Chrissie's thrush. The other points are all strong promoters of thrush, too, and are, fortunately, more easily reversible. What to do, though, about Don and the dancing? To recommend giving up sex and dancing would be unthinkable!

The ideas about the clothing after a dance work-out will help the perineum to cool down. We also chatted about changing from the leotard-demanding modern dance to any other sort of dance, and Chrissie went away muttering about flamenco and belly-dancing, both of which she quite likes and both of which do not require the wearing of leotards. She will give this some thought.

Sex is the other highly satisfying enjoyment in her life and if she cools the perineum afterwards with water from the bottle, doesn't have sex at all when thrush is next present, and has six months off the Pill, this problem area will also become controllable. The transmitting of thrush to and from Don to Chrissie and back again is absolutely controllable. The heat during sex still remains a hurdle.

All the bathing can be stopped and it is possible also to limit the showering. This is just willpower and life-revision not the changing of life itself, which is how one could regard the sex and dancing.

Chrissie is a reasonably typical modern young woman, active, sexual, food-conscious and hygiene-conscious. Sixty years ago her way of life would have been absolutely unthinkable, with its attendant poor sexual health, but we must all move with the times and its opportunities. The brake must go on, though, when health is under threat. Chrissie's is threatened. The activities which give her most enjoyment in life are proving the very causes of her problems and Chrissie is right to look closely at them.

Follow-up – September

The brakes have indeed been put on! Chrissie's first words on the phone were: 'It's been absolutely wonderful, no trouble of any sort since I came to see you in June. Thank you very much.'

Questioning revealed that she had worked towards two goals:

- removing sugar from her system
- reducing body heat

These have been achieved by stopping the tinned/bottled drinks like Diet Coke; no more Mars bars; reducing the fruit intake; stopping all alcohol and generally monitoring the amount of sugar that she ingests. Chrissie now says that she didn't realize quite how much sugar she had been taking in in the form of food and drink, but after thinking about it has reduced the level greatly to good effect.

Throughout the summer heat, Chrissie has continued dancing, but not in leotards. She has worn cotton shorts and thinks that in the winter she will return to the leotards because she is a serious devotee of modern dance needing to outline her body movements. Her routine after dancing will change instead. She will remove the leotards immediately and put on a long woolly skirt whilst her muscles cool slowly. Chrissie feels that for less devoted dancers and for simple keep-fit classes, substituting longjohns for the leotards might prove an acceptable and healthier alternative.

The four baths a week have been cut to one and the water is no longer scolding hot. She showers at other times. Pubic hair is regularly cut with scissors to ½ an inch in length. Every pair of jeans has been thrown out, and pants are now completely cotton, without a nylon base to the cotton gusset. Having successfully worked on all of this, Chrissie decided to remain on the mini Pill for contraceptive protection, and her relationship with Don is in excellent shape.

No thrush treatment has been necessary and neither has she felt the need to go for any vaginal swabs because, she says, 'I am completely well, there's no itching, no discharge and no symptoms after intercourse – even the eczema has completely gone. I think I was really just too hot within myself.'

Chrissie is preventing her thrush, and that is the only way to deal with this curse once you know that your body is prone to it. Her case highlights that modern living can be injurious to health and that the average female body requires more thoughtful care than many women give it.

CHAPTER FIVE

Mrs Meg Radment

Meg Radment, at a youthful-looking 49 years, has two main occupations in life. One: looking out for her brood of four children, one foster child, two lodgers and a visiting boyfriend. Two: working three afternoons a week in a Citizen's Advice Bureau in North London.

She was lucky in that having phoned for a counselling appointment one evening, I was able to fit her in the next morning owing to a cancelled appointment. She arrived wearing a Liberty-print blouse, beige corduroy skirt and new two-tone high heels. She was a bit out of breath because the lodger who had volunteered to babymind her four-year-old was still in bed at 10 o'clock when Meg needed to leave.

We had an hour and a half's counselling, which could possibly have run a few minutes longer – but she wanted to start work at the bureau on time if possible. She didn't need the bathroom and she didn't want a drink, so we got down to business straight away. She knew of me not only from the Citizen's Advice Bureau but also because she'd had my first book, *Understanding Cystitis*, in its first year of publication way back in 1972, and only this year had finally turned out the old U&I Club magazines!

Meg is mentally bright; she plays Bridge and controls her brood, she was good at answering questions and quick on the uptake of ideas. Her first three children came from her one and only marriage 1958–1973, her fourth child came from her next sexual partner, who lived with her, and now Terry, who doesn't live in, has been partnering her since 1982. Meg says that she wouldn't marry again for anything, nor have someone living in. Having an 'intermittent cup of tea' as she puts it, is absolutely ideal! Hers is a one-parent family.

Symptoms

Currently has cystitis – frequency and burning – but she is controlling it, following my first book, with water, painkillers and bicarbonate. This attack, as with all her others since 1958 – the date of her marriage – has started after intercourse a week ago. The number of attacks seems to depend upon the number of sex sessions in a short period of time, e.g. evening sex followed eight hours later by morning sex. An isolated sex session may not produce cystitis. She doesn't think that she has thrush but she might have. Thrush was found some years ago on a random vaginal swab but she hasn't been swabbed apart from that one occasion.

The perineum seems to be often sore and irritated, and again she can trace it back to 1958. She always used to have a discharge, but this has now lessened due to the menopause, which is just about over and has taken three years.

Urine cultures usually show E.Coli. When cultures aren't taken she is given antibiotics anyway.

Headaches – not migrainous but still painful. She can sometimes relate them to stress, sometimes not. She has had three in two months.

Ever since her first childbirth on 1961 she has had to bear down to help her bladder expel all its urine.

Meg has had three attacks of cystitis since Christmas, all related, she thinks, to sex.

Urological history

MSUs: When tested show E.Coli, and this latest one does.
IVP: None.
Cystoscopy: None.

She has never seen a urologist because she doesn't like being messed about and she therefore hasn't pressured for an appointment to see one.

Gynaecological history

Periods began aged 11 years. They were very light but dribbled away for a full seven days, much to her annoyance.

1974   An abortion followed by a D&C because she bled continuously. The gynaecologist followed up with two hormone injections and a course of hormone tablets. The bleeding stopped.

1976   D&C. This was suggested to facilitate the conception of her fourth child after three years without conceiving. It worked.

1981   Another D&C, again for continuous bleeding. This time it coincided with the start of menopausal symptoms.

Meg describes her gynaecologist as 'tame'. He goes along with any suggestions made, and between the two of them they have coped with her gynaecological problems pretty well. He's not been too hot though on thrush checks or vaginal swabs for the irritation. Thrush has been found once because it's only been investigated once. Meg has no discharge now since the menopause and is, if anything, dry.

Babies and pregnancies

One boy, 1961   Bad birth, heavy perineal tears, forceps, stitches. The doctor in attendance had just had an eye operation and was working with only one eye uncovered. After three nights in severe discomfort from poor stitches, Meg developed a pus-filled vaginal infection and had to be cleansed and swabbed with antibiotic solution and re-stitched.

One boy, 1963   Home delivery, no tearing, no stitching, excellent midwife.

One girl, 1967   Hospital delivery, lost three pints of blood and needed stitches.

One abortion, 1974   Foetus eight weeks.

One boy, 1978   Another bad delivery. Hospital again and a student midwife. The room was crammed with students, and despite all the attention Meg had fresh tears and heavy stitching.

One abortion, 1979   Amniocentesis performed at 21 weeks showed a severely malformed foetus which could not possibly survive, so it was removed by caesarian section.

One foster child   Now three years old and on long term fostering.
  Meg has always done short term fostering.

Contraception

It has mostly been the dutch cap together with Orthogynol spermicidal jelly since 1958. One year on the Pill made no difference to
the sexual cystitis, nor does withdrawal, which has also been used
often. No contraception has been used for a year and Meg firmly
'feels' that she is no longer fertile.

Sex

Attacks of cystitis occurred with all three partners, probably least
with the husband because he was 'indifferent' to sexual desire. Sex
with Terry is sporadic now because Meg is absolutely fed up with
the expectation of cystitis. In their first year of being partners Meg
lubricated better, probably because of their 'chemistry' and probably
because the vagina was not fully involved in the onset of the
menopause.

Sex lasts about half an hour or so. In the last two years with
sporadic sex, Terry has usually ejaculated with ease in the evening
sex session, meaning that Meg's vagina has had less rubbing and
friction. A second session later on means that he takes longer to
ejaculate and Meg puts up with extra rubbing on a previously swollen
vagina.

KY Jelly is used but the second sexual partner, who lived in,
didn't like KY so Meg got out of the habit of using it in dollops.
She only uses a smear.

She passes urine after sex, but after a second session finds that
she has no urine in her bladder to pass. She does wash after sex,
but sits on the edge of the bidet – which is plugged up – and she
slooshes water up onto her perineum. She does not clean sexual
liquids out of the vagina nor does she wash before intercourse.

The act of intercourse seems comfortable except in any second
session and penetration is easy. Meg enjoys sex but is naturally a
little reticent because of the fear of cystitis. Since reading my first
book in 1972, cystitis has lessened in severity and fear because she
can tame it by initiating water and bicarbonate management straight
away.

Clothing

This is all wrong! She wears tights, tight jeans, trousers, cotton pants laundered with the daily wash and forced by the jeans seam onto the tender urethral/vaginal skin.

General health

Meg is energetic and feels well. Her family has no major health-problem history. She has rectal skin tabs caused by the pregnancies and births.

Fluid intake

Not too bad but could improve a little. The daily intake is about 4–5 pints a day except when she is dealing with an attack of cystitis. There is no sign of acidity and twingeing.

Diet

Doesn't come into this case.

My suggestions (chronologically put down at counselling):

1 Can you relate headaches to changes in urinary output/retention?
2 Keep a fluid balance chart for one week.
3 Old scars from the birth tears can harbour bacteria and respond badly to careless intercourse.
4 No more tights, trousers or jeans.
5 Undies MUST be boiled, not put in the launderette with the other wash. This alone may be causing the irritation.
6 Don't ever use that bidet again. You are not removing E.Coli, you are helping it to spread!
7 Wash as I have demonstrated with the bottle method after a stool and after sex.
8 Rectal skin tabs harbour E. Coli. The bottle-washing method, together with your free hand and the soapy water cleansing between the tabs, will effectively remove faecal material.
9 I gave the name of a gynaecologist for:
(a) hormone assessment – dry skin, irritation, menopause.

(b) scar assessment – how delicate are these scars and is one too close to the rectal orifice?

(c) vaginal/cervical assessment and swabs – thrush particularly.

10 Use LOTS of KY Jelly before and during intercourse. A smear is not enough to pad the vagina and reduce the risk of bruising.

11 Use it especially in any second sex session.

12 Always keep the bladder urine level reasonable. Have a glass of water around 9.30 each night and again after sex.

13 The first year with Terry was probably better lubricated. After three years, plus ageing skin due to the menopause, dryness will now be more likely.

14 Once you and Terry know that attacks of cystitis after sex are highly unlikely due to better hygiene and the physical feel of the KY Jelly padding, his need for two sessions close together may recede and with that, the likelihood of bruising and soreness.

15 A new pattern of twice/thrice weekly sex with good intervals may emerge.

16 You have very sensitive skin.

17 Lack of hormones, which lower during the menopause, are a common cause of dryness in women over 45. The perineal/vaginal skin becomes irritable and less able to ward off infections.

18 The cap could have been an additional cause of sexual cystitis over the years, but symptoms persist despite over a year without using the cap.

19 Even though you have not seen a urologist, and I don't even now think that is necessary, I still don't feel that you have a urological reason for this cystitis. Your attacks clearly follow sex and you have no bladder symptoms in between actual attacks.

20 If the bladder, which you say needs pressure to completely empty, was harbouring bacteria, you would be in pain, with impromptu fevers and general malaise. You are not in such a state.

My comments

Dealing with 19 and 20 first. The general practitioner would also appear to agree with me since in the 26 years that Meg has had her symptoms, he has not referred her for a kidney X-ray, cystoscopy or even to a urologist. Some would disagree vehemently with this and say that such investigations could be vital. Experience shows that IVPs and cystoscopies are negative in cystitis related to intercourse.

The GP has saved NHS time and money and also removed the likelihood of damage by an operation-happy urologist. Meg has been spared the rigours of dilatation and urological intervention. On this she is lucky.

Luck has also been with her in that belonging all those years ago to the old U&I Club and reading my early book she has been able for fifteen years to contain her bad symptoms with self-help. Although cystitis has continued, mostly due to inaccurate application of the rules in my book, she has not feared cystitis. She has, quite naturally, been upset that she hasn't managed to stop it altogether.

This pressure that she has to exert in order to pass all her urine is not accompanied by any pain, nor is the act of micturition uncomfortable; so, although, at first, I wondered whether she is retaining bacteria-laden urine, I decided against this. Meg is free of all symptoms when undergoing a spell without sex. She does not have a temperalture, nor feel ill, nor does she experience a pain in the bladder/pelvic region *during* intercourse. Whatever happened to the bladder upon the birth of her first child has mercifully not added to the attacks of cystitis.

A micturating cystogram may show muscular ineptitude of some sort following a birth tear but, whatever it is, her bladder and urethra are not being affected by it in terms of distress or real malfunction.

Just in case the fluid intake does not match the urine output, and as an additional check to any occasional mild water-retention, I told Meg how to keep a fluid intake chart.

For one week drink all your drinks from one specific cup or mug. Fill whatever mug you have chosen with tapwater and pour it off into a measuring jug. Note how much it holds, e.g. 6 fluid ounces.

Make a seven day chart:

Mon		Tues		Wed		Thurs		Fri		Sat		Sun	
in	out	in	out	in	out	in	out	in	out	in	out	in	out
a.m.		a.m.		a.m.		a.m.		a.m.		a.m.		a.m.	
3		2											
1	2	3											
p.m.		p.m.		p.m.		p.m.		p.m.		p.m.		p.m.	
4	1	5											
8	3	10											

Then add up the weekly total of in: out:

The 'in' is measured by mug/cupfuls, e.g. 8 mug/cupfuls on Monday.

The 'out' is measured into a measuring jug by the ounce/pint, e.g. 3 pints on Monday.

You will probably pass more urine in the first act of micturition each morning so by the *end* of the week you may have balanced up roughly but you may not balance the 'in' against the 'out' each day. For the daily 'in' measurement in ounces/pints you must multiply 8 mug/cupfuls by what you have previously ascertained that it holds, e.g.,
   6 fluid ounces × 8 mug/cupfuls (for the Monday example)
   6 fluid ounces × 60 mug/cupfuls (for the week's total)

You can do this for a whole month, if you like, to take into account the build-up to a period, the period itself and the rest of the month. Only a rough guide is required because other factors like thirst, salt intake, sweating etc., will be having individual daily effects.

   External birth scars are a problem for many women. The seam of skin that runs along the uppermost join of both sides of the perineum and links all three openings has to be elastic and with good muscle tone. A scar does not have muscle tone and is easily nicked or bruised. Such scars can be heavily affected by intercourse, foreplay, constipation and straining, any further childbirth, bicycle rides, swimming, vaginal and perineal infections, investigative gynae-cological work and probably a host of other things from individual life-styles.

To try to compensate for the scar's lack of elasticity, any help you can give to the remaining unscarred section of muscle should be attempted. Remembering to pull the pelvis and perineum up whenever an opportune moment arises can help. It's enjoyable during intercourse to grip your partner's penis with the vaginal muscles. It's no effort to do one or more of the simple exercises in my other book whilst lying in bed and it's not inconvenient to pull up two or three times *once you have passed* all urine and you're still sitting on the loo. Pulling up and tilting the hips backwards whilst you walk is another way of toning the pelvic support and strengthening scarred muscles.

Meg had sexual cystitis for three years prior to her first childbirth and E.Coli was always found in her urine. I did not ask her to show me how she washed in detail. It was enough to hear the words 'plugged up bidet', and I knew that even before ever using that bidet, which she's done for many years, she has a poor idea of hygiene and has never effectively removed E.Coli from her perineum. The rectal skin tabs and the perineal birth scars will all harbour germs from faecal material.

In intercourse, the E.Coli from this ineffective hygiene will be massaged into Meg's urethra by the rubbing going on next door in the vagina. This is the classic 'honeymoon' cystitis. This is the old 'playground too close to the sewage farm' joke so beloved of medical personnel. Well, you can't stop the rubbing and massaging move-ments of sex and neither can you eradicate E.Coli from its natural habitat, the bowels; so you *must* remove the 'travelling' aspect of E.Coli between the bowels and the bladder opening. E.Coli adores warm, mildly acidic bladder urine. It does not like over-acid urine (neither do the bladder nerve-endings!) nor dilute alkaline urine. It is up to the patient to confine her own E.Coli *within* the bowels and maintain a bacteria-free rectal orifice.

In the bottle-washing method, the hand not holding the bottle is vital in removing soapy liquid from the rectal orifice, even more so if skin tabs and haemorrhoids are there. Your hand and fingers must wriggle around between the tabs to aid the rinsing process whilst the warm water from the bottle is flowing.

Personally speaking, it is this simple, so simple process that has kept me completely free from cystitis. Remember, my first five years of marriage was all E.Coli cystitis. No more!

On the bottom line – pardon the pun again! – Meg is still a honeymoon cystitis victim even after all these years. Despite all the other nineteen points of my suggestions to her, she may respond fast to the washing and never again have a true E.Coli bladder infection following intercourse. We'll see.

She mentioned early that she does pass urine after sex but can't do so if a second session happens. She hadn't thought to drink more water to compensate or even to drink after the first session in preparation for a possible second. This she will now start to do, and she should be able to pass urine after any act of intercourse at whatever time of the day or night it takes place.

Bruising and trauma of the cervix, vagina and perineum can be regarded as probable if soreness and a swollen feeling seem to start right after intercourse. Counteracting this is as easy as putting lots of KY Jelly at the entrance to the vagina and also stroking the penis with a nice sticky hand. He doesn't have to know that you're doing it for any other reason than *his* pleasure! A well-lubricated woman is an added excitement to a man – it has always been so since Adam, and actually it's my opinion that Eve didn't offer him an apple. I think she offered him a tube of KY Jelly!

Lubrication is a padding and an aid to elasticity of the vagina. KY acts psychologically, not just to the man, but also to a tired, tense woman. She knows that by protecting her vagina she is also protecting her bladder and she relaxes into the enjoyment.

In all these years Meg has used the diaphragm or dutch cap as her main contraceptive. Had she stopped cystitis whilst on the Pill, or stopped cystitis altogether last year when she stopped using the cap, I'd say that she belonged to that band of women whose cervixes are battered in sex by the movement of the cap and its hard rim. But this wasn't the case. Possibly some of her cystitis attacks have been due to the cap, but we can't categorically prove it from what Meg has said because she continues to have E.Coli bladder infections after sexual intercourse *without* the cap.

Cool water after each act of intercourse poured from the bottle down the perineum to reduce swollen tissues must in turn be abetted by hooking out sexual liquids from the vagina with your long finger.

Otherwise these liquids can go stale, harbour any stray bacteria and crack, a little like candlegrease does when it's dried out, leaving your skin feeling sore. Don't *sit* in cool water, you must *pour* it from front to back after you've passed urine and while you are still on the loo, not forgetting to finger-clean the perineum whilst the water is flowing from the bottle.

If Terry can understand that Meg may from now on be cystitis-free and that sex doesn't have to be sporadic, he may manage on single sex sessions at night two or three times a week. Morning sex means for Meg that her vagina is denied a good night's rest. If she has been getting up after morning sex, putting on chemically contaminated underwear, air-restricting tights and close-fitting jeans, her perineum will have remained swollen and bruised; her bladder will not be emptied with a good dilute urinary flow until after the breakfast drinks have gone through; and all in all, things couldn't be much worse.

The right clothing for victims of thrush and cystitis is very important. The perineum was designed for maximum air access in order to keep cool and dry and avoid helping bacteria to thrive. Tight or close-fitting clothing restricts air access and encourages sweating. Jean seams bruise the inner labia and the vulva (where the front two openings meet) and also prevent air from cooling the skin. It's no good pouring water from the bottle down the perineum to cool it if you then go and stop air from continuing this cooling. Victims should wear skirts, stockings and belts, cotton undies and mixture petticoats. Baggies and low-crotched culottes are all right; leotards and body stockings are not.

Thrush may be present. It's not obvious to Meg, but since she didn't know that she had it on the one swab that showed it, she may have it semi-permanently in a mild form. Since I feel that the gynaecologist ought to have a check on things like menopausal hormone levels he might as well, and would anyway, look for thrush on his swabs.

He may also find that the poor stitching of that half-blind gynaecologist in 1961 is aggravating the bruising during intercourse. Perhaps, even though Meg says sex is comfortable, there is a small area of vaginal stricture which could be eased.

Meg may turn out to be complicated and not respond quickly to my suggestions. After all, she's had cystitis since 1958. But she does, fortunately, seem to recover well in between attacks and I have every hope that the self-help procedures for sex plus the bottle-washing after a stool will combine to do the trick.

I have maintained for many years that cystitis related to intercourse is entirely preventable and manageable. That doesn't mean to say that an occasional attack won't occur, but it does mean that the victim will be more likely to know why and pull her socks up quickly!

Follow-up

Meg has carefully changed the past routines, giving thought and time to them. She uses the bottle-washing method, of course, but personally finds it easier to manipulate when sitting on the bidet not the lavatory. She only sits on the bidet to rinse off with the bottle; she does not use the equipment itself for washing and rinsing, so I don't mind her adaptation.

The fluid-intake chart has not been kept, largely because she's been busily assisting an ailing daughter who has contracted glandular fever – but also because everything else seems to be working well.

She hasn't been to see the specialist with reference to hormone evaluation for the same reasons, and feels that this is something which she can hold in reserve.

Sexual intercourse has taken place and it has not brought on cystitis or twingeing. The new tips and spacing of sessions appear to have worked.

As Meg says, 'I may well relapse occasionally in the future, but for now I feel very confident and should be able to work out the reason for any relapse if it ever happens.'

So far, so good and simple. An intelligent use of the counselling, and we hope that all will remain well for many years to come.

CHAPTER SIX

Mrs June Sharott and Ben

Mrs June Sharott, aged 41, lives in Rotherham with her husband Ben. She and a girlfriend came down to London to combine the counselling with some Oxford Street shopping. The girlfriend elected to read the paper and watch something on television elsewhere in the house whilst Mrs Sharott and I got down to business.

She was attractively dressed in a matching crêpe dress and high-heeled shoes, altogether presenting herself as someone with an interest in smartness. Standing somewhere between 5 foot 3 and 5 foot 6, she was not slim but probably around a size 14.

She had left school at sixteen desperate to dance, and had slowly built up a thriving dance school – ballet, modern and tap – in which she herself taught for 24 years. In 1980 she began to take on extra work as an entertainments agent booking artists to appear in clubs on the Midlands or Northern circuits. These clubs vary from small to huge memberships, and many of our famous variety acts go through their doors en route to further successes.

June began to enjoy this greatly and has become highly regarded both by the artists and the club managers, so that each night of the week – Sundays are spent in bed recovering – she stands in the bars doing business with managers of different clubs and spotting new talents. This necessitates much social drinking, which, in such places, lays great emphasis on alcohol.

With this new venture becoming very profitable, she finally decided after 24 years to sell her dancing school and become a full time artists' agent. By 1983, she had severed all teaching connections and settled into the night life of the clubs. Daytime is divided between sleeping late, then getting on the telephone or writing letters, and travelling later to one or more club appointments each evening.

Ben and June have been very happily married since their early twenties. He has discovered and developed a pleasant nightclub voice and sings as vocalist a couple of nights a week, but his main work is as a scaffolder (up high buildings) five days a week, 9–5. He leads a high old life!

June had travelled all the way to see me, as so many do, in abject desperation, quite unable to see an end to her symptoms.

Symptoms

Just one – vaginal thrush so severe that it was down the inside of her thighs. Other symptoms were classic – intense irritation, curdy discharge and perineal redness, all driving her crazy. She had not been clear of it since it started in 1980 and had taken many appropriate courses of treatment. Oral medication had never been prescribed, only local vaginal pessaries or cream.

Urological history

None – no trouble.

Gynaecological history

Her periods began at 14 and were very heavy and extremely painful. The first three days each month were spent in bed, right through until the year that her first baby was born when she was 23.
No D&Cs (Dilatation and Curettage)
Childhood polio had seemingly left little trouble, until June found on marrying that full penetration was impossible. When she became pregnant, the doctor pronounced it an 'Act of God' because examination showed a displaced bone brought about by the polio. This offending obstacle was removed during the birth of her first child.

Sex

No penetration possible until bone removed in 1965. Penetration was possible thereafter and it would be frequent, enjoyable and pain-free now exccpt for the thrush.

Contraception

After the first baby, June went on the Pill for two years, but after the second baby in 1968, Ben had a vasectomy.

Babies

One girl, born 1965   Appalling birth, general anaesthetic but peri-
neal delivery because of bone complication. Many stitches.
One girl, born 1968   Vaginal delivery with forceps and episiotomy.
Dreadful birth and lots more stitches.
One boy   Adopted at six years old.

General

Health, apart from thrush, is good, but she feels very tired. She
never needs to take antibiotics.

Clothing

She wears cotton underwear, stockings and suspenders. No jeans.

Hygiene

As with many thrush sufferers she feels that she must bath frequently
– twice a day.

Liquid intake

Normal except for alcohol and lots of it each evening.

Ben

Has excessive stomach and bowel wind with rectal irritation.

My suggestions

1   The major cause of June's thrush is the alcohol each night.
   Alcohol converts to sugar and thrush thrives in a sugar
   medium. Stop the alcohol.
2   Drink any unsweetened mineral water like Perrier, Evian,
   soda or tonic instead.
3   Ben obviously has thrush, too.
4   BOTH of you are to go in future to any VD/genito-urinary
   clinic for checks whenever necessary. These clinics have
   microscopes and give immediate accurate diagnosis plus free
   treatment.
5   Go to a clinic now and return at the end of treatment for a
   clearance check.

6   Strongly request Nystatin oral tablets both for you and Ben.
7   Whenever Ben has antibiotics, he should take Nystatin tablets as prevention of thrush.
8   Anti-fungal pessaries must be inserted as high as the cervix, which can only be done when lying flat on your back. If they don't slide easily, use some KY Jelly on the pessary tip.
9   Don't have intercourse when thrush is present or suspected in either partner. Intercourse will aggravate it and your partner can catch thrush.
10 For now – no sex for the next two weeks and then use a sheath for a week.
11 Since thrush is worse in hot weather, wear cool clothes and keep cool. Go without underwear whenever possible; long clothes can make this possible during the day.
12 Avoid sugary foods and soft drinks like cola.
13 No more baths. Have stand-up washes for two months and use the bottle method for washing the perineum.
14 How about a blood test for anaemia?
15 Severe candida (thrush) can be regarded as an allergic reaction (e.g. an allergy to the alcohol). With the immune system desperately trying to cope with the candida, lethargy, often another symptom of thrush, can result.

My comments

The new job involving heavy social drinking began in 1980; so did thrush. June didn't have thrush before this, not even when she went on the Pill briefly. One has to assume and connect the high alcohol intake with thrush.

To June's way of looking at things, the drinking *is* the job and although she recognized it as the cause of her continuous trouble, she was most reluctant to stop. She had a difficult choice to make:
1   Give up the drinking and stop thrush
2   Keep thrush and carry on drinking
The pressures put on her each night by barmen, business men and artists to 'have a drink', 'have another, go on', 'what'll it be?' were almost insurmountable, and she thought that they would laugh at her if she desisted or asked for mineral water. Indeed, I realized that these people could be very insistent, but still put it to her that once in a glass with lemon and ice, plain water looks just like a gin

and tonic. A quiet word with the barman might help, or telling the roundsman about having a very real allergy to alcohol.

Putting it ruthlessly, she had to give up alcohol somehow!

Ben, although a thoroughly helpful and kindly husband, might not like forgoing sex for the duration of treatment; nor might he be, like so many men, keen to be genitally examined. Men don't have babies and aren't used to being examined as women are. This, too, June had to explain and hope for cooperation.

Some doctors don't like prescribing oral Nystatin, but with Ben's thrush being in the gut and bowels, he certainly had to have oral treatment. June needed it, too, because she has had continuous trouble now for some years. So another discussion with a not too helpful doctor had to be gone through.

All in all there were difficulties.

Follow-up

June came to see me in February. I followed up in July. On leaving me she had a three-week course of anti-fungal treatment, orally and locally. She gave up alcohol totally and helped herself still further by joining a slimmers' club. They don't allow alcohol. She was very clever to boost her confidence and moral support in this way. She admits to having started bathing again and that, in combination with hot weather last week, has caused her first attack of thrush since February. She has instantly stopped the baths, taken off the underwear and had a week of oral Nystatin and Canesten pessaries. All symptoms have gone.

She has passed the book around and says that the best train journey she ever took was to London to see me. This woman now fully understands thrush. Like everyone, she will probably remain prone to it but she has amply proved for herself the helpfulness of prevention so she has overcome it. Any attack of thrush must be treated with conventional medications, it also has to be prevented according to the individual patient's life-style. A great success story, this one!

CHAPTER SEVEN

Mrs Wendy Blokkers and Theo

It was Wendy Blokkers' mother who first approached me by telephone for help for her daughter. She felt that Wendy, although she had read one of my books some months previously, was not getting anywhere with conventional treatment and was steadily getting worse. In fact, she was apparently so unwell that travelling was extremely difficult and the girl needed her mother to drive her down from Cheshire. After three abortive attempts to come, I asked whether the girl could not travel by train to see me herself, and only then did Wendy ring me for the first time.

Another date was fixed and kept. Her young husband, Theo, 28 years old and working with a firm of accountants, had taken the day off to drive his wife to see me, and it later transpired, also to a gynaecologist recommended by a friend. Wendy is 25 and looks 17. She used to work as a typist until her marriage in mid-1982, but health problems have since forced her to stop. Just before coming to see me she had been persuaded to take a small part-time secretarial job to take her mind off things. In the first three weeks of this new job she has had to take two days off already, and the day of the counselling was the third.

Wendy could have walked off the film set of John Travolta's *Summer Nights*. She wore a blouse and skirt and sandals. Her brown hair was shoulder-length and neatly brushed back, and she wore very little make-up. She looked soft, unworldly and radiated a need for protection. Both mother and husband provided this, as far as I could tell.

She had recently begun an hour of keep-fit a week to try to regain some of her lost zest, but her ability to enjoy a good walk was still impaired. Musical and sensitive, she played both violin and piano with a degree of skill, and so did Theo.

Theo had elected to sit in on the counselling and, as is often the case, proved most helpful. I gave him my normal armchair and seated myself behind the desk.

Symptoms

Cystitis with blood, pain, frequency, high temperature and vomiting. Often the temperature was by itself or accompanied by a feeling of general malaise. Vaginal discharges were also a frequent factor, the last one being in April and showing streptococci on the swab result. Mild sore throat, often tired, diarrhoea since she was 13, which was always worse during a period. Perineal soreness upwards and in. The cystitis had occurred seven times in the first year of marriage and had been consistently severe, with all the other symptoms ever since – two years.

Urological history

Mid-stream urine tests: Lots and always infected. As with so many women, Wendy never asked the name of the bacteria, nor was this vital information volunteered.

Antibiotics: Septrin and others. Lots of courses.

Intravenous pyelogram: One, negative.

Cystoscopy: One, negative but showing inflammation of bladder lining.

Urethral Dilatation: One, December 1983. No improvement (usually the case).

Plenty of hospital and GP involvement.

Gynaecological history

Periods began aged 14 and were sporadic with great pain and vomiting for four years. At 18 she was put on the Pill for two years and taken off because of headaches. A year later the periods were back to being awful. A lower-dosage oestrogen Pill was then tried, but some breakthrough bleeding began and with two further experiments with other Pills and a renewal of the headaches the Pill generally was abandoned.

No D&Cs.

Babies and pregnancies

None.

Sex

Wendy is very dry, tense and finds intercourse painful because of the multitude of symptoms. Intercourse has occurred twice between January and March.

General health

She has never had an operation except those mentioned in the urological history. There are obvious hormone problems as in the period and Pill histories. Diarrhoea is a daily factor which commenced at puberty. One of Wendy's grandmothers was diabetic.

Self-help

She has read my books and says that she is following my routines.

Food and liquid intake

Reasonably all right, but in view of the presence of so many positive bacterial counts both on vaginal and urethral cultures, food and liquid intake is largely irrelevant.

Clothing

She wears stockings and suspenders, no jeans or trousers, and, again, this section is irrelevant.

Hygiene

Appalling! Upstairs in my bathroom checking out Wendy's insistence that she is following the instructions for washing in my book, such a dreadful tale came out that it became all too obvious how big a part this was playing in her continuous trouble. Several times a day Wendy was sitting back to front on a bidet and washing loose diarrhoea forward and into the vagina. Hence the constant streptococci in the vaginal swab. Before 1983, she didn't wash at all. The chapter in my book on washing had, contrary to her accounts, been flagrantly disobeyed.

My suggestions

1 Never use a bidet. It can be extremely dangerous.
2 Revise, as of today, the hygiene procedure and follow it exactly as demonstrated and written about in my book.
3 Check for thrush today and regularly because of the heavy antibiotics taken so far.
4 Take the course of Augmentin prescribed for the latest vaginal streptococci infection diagnosed yesterday again.
5 How about trying a progestagen-based contraceptive pill such as Nordette by Wyeth Pharmaceuticals of West Germany?
6 ASK the name of any bacteria found in any urine specimen. Don't leave the consulting room until you do know!
7 A hormone check would be helpful. The periods and Pill history, the fact that all symptoms worsen near a period, the diarrhoea since puberty, can all point to a hormone malfunction.
8 Always ask for Nystatin tablets and pessaries if you have to take any further antibiotics.
9 When intercourse is resumed after clearance tests on the vagina and when you appear to be comfortably free of symptoms, use lots of KY Jelly to aid lubrication and guard against vaginal bruising.
10 I wonder whether there are any food allergies which might be causing the diarrhoea?
11 I gave the name of the York Alternative Medical Practice, 4 Museum Street, York, telephone: 0904 52378, for allergy testing.
12 Wendy's tonsils are still in. It's worth checking if and what bacteria are present there, in view of her sore throats, and whether they match any bacteria found in urine samples. The sore throats could also be associated with allergies.

My comments

There is no doubt at all in my mind that Wendy's gullibility and ignorance in using the bidet, and prior to that not washing at all, are the causes of her downfall. Although she couldn't name her urinary bacteria, I would have bet a large sum of money on it being E.Coli and/or streptococci from her bowels.

This daily and repetitious transfer of bacteria to both urethra and vagina would account for the malaise, high fevers and sore throats. To have had intercourse – Theo's impatience with Wendy showed up during our bathroom session – under such infected conditions could only have caused huge reactions in the vagina and urethra.

The diarrhoea two or three times a day was an extra hazard, especially since it was never cleared away, and it would be interesting to know whether the hormone levels are responsible or whether there are any food allergies. Personally, I'd go for the hormone levels in her case. Women with sensitive hormone levels before motherhood do sometimes pull round after having their first baby, and as most women will tell you, our bowels and urinary output undergo changes in their normal routines near or during a period. This is hormonal.

Washing after intercourse was also discussed, demonstrated and reasoned out for her, so together with the help of KY Jelly, I see no reason at present to find anything else in the way of a happy sex life. Theo deserves one after all this!

Of course, such a start to sex must have taken a toll not only on the relationship, but also on the delicate skin of the genital area. It will need much correct cosseting for many months to recover and stabilize.

I'm afraid that I almost became belligerent in my attempts to get it through to her that she and she alone was responsible for all these infections and, having had one of my books, she really had no excuse either. The medical profession cannot prevent vaginal and urethral infections; they can only treat those shown to be present. Only Wendy can prevent her bowels from causing ill health in her body. I wonder what the friend's gynaecologist had to say after the pair left me.

Follow-up – July

The London gynaecologist recommended by the friend found no thrush and said that he felt the vaginal opening was too small, so recommended an enlargement – vaginal dilation. Wendy's reaction was to discount this idea, and she agreed with me that Theo could penetrate her perfectly easily in size. The dryness in two subsequent attempts at intercourse was much helped by the KY Jelly, which Wendy had used copiously.

The bidet has not been used even once, Wendy assured me, and apart from one small dose of cystitis for unknown reasons, so far, there have been no more vaginal infections. The washing is now well revised and settled as an essential routine following any kind of bowel movement.

Wendy has not taken my advice on seeking investigations into the hormones. Perhaps on my résumé notes for her to take with her, I didn't really hammer it home hard enough for her to understand. The local gynaecologist in Cheshire scorned the idea of investigating them, and I dare say Wendy didn't pursue it. She hasn't done her own experiment with Nordette or requested it from her GP, so absolutely no headway has been undertaken in this very important gap.

Neither has she followed up my suggestion to ascertain the presence of any allergies which may be another cause of her constant daily diarrhoea.

Instead, she has kept a long-held appointment with another urologist. This man has advised that she needs the following:

A urothrometry
A urethral cystometry
A urethral function study
A cysto-urothroscopy

Wendy reckons this is all a bit high-flung, and in discussion with me has decided to hold it in reserve for about three months.

There are no current infections anywhere, and my guess is that short of carelessness there never will be any more, but Wendy is now left with a feeling that something is still not quite right! Her bladder still feels sensitive and two gentle sessions with intercourse have still been a bit sore, even though the KY Jelly was 'fantastic' and no infections resulted.

I suggested that after these traumas the whole region just needed time to continue its recovery. It has undergone a very nasty two years. To reduce still further any bladder sensitivity, I recommended a level teaspoonful of bicarbonate of soda each night before bed for

10 days and warned her off the wonderful soft fruit which we are currently enjoying!

I also suggested that she and Theo make a regular date to have intercourse, and I pointed out the old adage 'lose it or use it'! The KY and the cool water with lots of finger foreplay will relax the vagina and increase the desires.

I pressed again on the hormone and allergy levels, citing once more the reasons why I felt them necessary. It also needed to be explained that these tests are done off blood samples and nothing more alarming than that. Wendy seemed much reassured and will discuss them with Theo tonight. Since her Cheshire gynaecologist laughed at the thought of hormone investigations, I gave the name of a gynaecologist in London whom I know to be good in this field. I must stress that many gynaecologists do work in this field all over the country but Wendy is unlucky in hers.

I also reminded her that previous urological investigations and treatment had proved negative. It seems to me that further work up that channel would have a similar outcome, and this suggests that she leaves well alone.

Further follow-up – September

Wendy and Theo are to move to London for his new job in six weeks' time. This has led her to continue seeing her Cheshire gynaecologist 'because he keeps on giving me the pills – Septrin – even though he and the treatment aren't helping'! When they arrive in London, she will see my recommended gynaecologist. Although symptoms aren't so severe and she is keeping up with her part-time job, the vagina and urethra have still shown coliform and mixed infections on four occasions. The last occasion occurred only on a routine check by the gynaecologist; Wendy was not actually having an attack of cystitis but he found bacteria in the routine samples. I strongly suspect that she is still just not washing properly, even though she is adamant that she is washing exactly as I showed. The last attack resulted from not washing at all after a bowel movement whilst on a trip to Stratford-on-Avon. Intercourse did not occur later, she says, and, indeed, it has only happened once in the last four months.

It transpires that Theo has now washed his hands of her troubles, and who can blame him – I can sympathize. I warned her that she'll have no marriage soon and she agreed – so blandly and still in the same little-girl voice that one can only suppose that she isn't suffering *that* badly or she would stop at nothing to finish this sad state of affairs.

I pushed her hard on the hygiene again and said some strong words about the failure to seek better medical help, but this girl has no spunk, no fight in her. It may be months now before she actually rings up my suggested gynaecologist. She first saw me on 2 May, and it is now 12 September, with no headway having been made. At least the high fevers, malaise and using that bidet have stopped but the rest of it is very disappointing. This girl should by now be completely well.

CHAPTER EIGHT

Mrs Dawn Carling

Mrs Carling's doctor had reckoned that what she really needed was some self-help since everything that had so far been done to her by his profession had failed to resolve the problem; indeed, she has steadily worsened and to date has had to take the last twelve months off work.

At 51 years old, she is a cook/supervisor for Staffordshire County Council education department. They have paid her salary steadfastly during these past twelve months and, prior to that, over an eight-year period much interrupted by the same symptoms. Next week she has to go before a medical board to assess her condition and advise the school board of her future fitness for work.

If she is proved unfit and unlikely to work again, they will have to pension her off and employ a new full-time person to fill her job vacancy. Dawn loved her work and indeed arrived looking every inch the organized character that she was. Not tall, about 5 foot 3, in black high heels with a lovely pale green tailored tweed suit and cream blouse, she was accompanied by her tall blonde daughter-in-law and small grandchild.

For the 1½ hours of our counselling session the daughter-in-law and grandchild watched television in another part of the house and went out for a walk.

The three of them had come down to London from the Midlands on away day train tickets and, after leaving me, were going to say a brief hello to Oxford Street and enjoy a nice meal before taking a train home at 7.15 p.m.

Gregory, Dawn's husband and partner in their 30-year marriage, has seen hard times of late. His own building firm has lost its 30 or so employees, and now Gregory contracts-out on large commitments or takes on temporary labour as and when needed. Otherwise he works entirely on his own. He loves golf, fishing and snooker, and if Dawn had not been feeling so ill she would be golfing with him. Their only child, Jim, is a professional golfer and the family enjoy this mutual interest.

So here is a woman who doesn't look well, whose entire life is in a state of suspension, whose career and marital relationship have been upended, and who is searching, as she says, for the person or persons 'I must inevitably find who will make me well again'. Staffordshire education department, whose bills are met by rate-payers, have been forced to pay a double salary for the one job – Dawn plus her temporary replacement; Dawn has been paying too in pain, frustration, countless visits to doctor and hospital, private gynaecological care; and the beleaguered National Health Service has spent thousands of pounds on her in terms of doctor-time, antibiotics and other drugs, hospital admission and operations, urological tests.

And she is no better. She is worse!

AND THE COUNTRY IS OVER TWENTY THOUSAND POUNDS WORSE OFF!

Symptoms

Severe perineal irritation, all orifices particularly, and she scratches. Yesterday was bad; today the pressure is off. She feels sore and swollen inside, and has to get up frequently during the night to pass urine. There is bad backache and nasty pelvic pain which seem to match with one another; today is not too bad. There has never been a report of thrush or any other bacterial invasion on swabs.

Urine tests show bacteria but she has never asked what it was or is and she has never been told. This is a great hindrance to my efforts in the counselling session. When her GP told her to contact me he also mentioned hygiene, and with that as my only clue, I am going to have to assume, probably wrongly, that it's E.Coli. I hate assuming anything so important, but E.Coli is so common that it is probably the safest of the bets. This has all been going on for seven or eight years from age 43 in 1976. The visit last week to the VD unit, which I had suggested on the phone when our counselling was fixed, had given an all-clear on their standard tests.

So it's bladder infections – supposedly E.Coli – great soreness and irritation, pelvic pain and backache.

Urological history

MSUs   Lots! Sometimes with unnamed infection and
   sometimes with something else but, again, not revealed.
Micturating Cystogram: 1981. Negative
Intravenous pyelogram: 1981. Negative
Cystoscopy: Three, *all negative* between 1981 and 1984. Two
   were NHS, one private.
Dilatations of the urethra: Two
Bladder stretches: Three

Dawn has no idea why they were done and unquestioningly accepted everything. She is absolutely furious with the urological treatment, knowing now the awful truth that her symptoms are still with her. After one negative IVP, one negative cystogram and three negative cystoscopies, five further operations were performed on her! She does not have interstitial cystitis.

Gynaecological history

Periods began aged 14 years and were very painful but not heavy. Upon her marriage the pain went and periods became trouble-free.
Vaginal swabs – all negative.
Last year the private gynaecologist gave a single month's course of Premarin, a hormone preparation. At the end of that month there was no follow-up, no discussion nor further courses. On 22 August this year, the general practitioner prescribed a course of Dinoestrol vaginal hormone cream, and Dawn thinks she remembers, since it wasn't that long ago, feeling slightly less sore then and also on the Premarin.
No D&Cs.
Age 17 she had a severe fall down the stairs and was hospitalized for two weeks, which included perineal surgery on a long tear in the labia minora – that fold of skin which lies beneath the two external labia which are covered in pubic hair.
In 1969, fifteen years ago, a large benign tumour was found in the uterus; also a cyst on the right ovary. Both organs were removed. She was 36.

Babies

One boy – born 1954, and on a post-natal check-up an unhealed vaginal tear was discovered, locally anaesthetized and stitched.

Contraception

Dawn began married life using a dutch cap and spermicidal cream but hated all the messiness, so she and Gregory decided to stick on withdrawal. Following the hysterectomy there was no need for any contraception.

Sex

Prior to the last nine years intercourse was twice weekly or so. Within the last nine years the rate went down by a half, and as the vaginal sorenesses increased she finally ended up in another bedroom and has been there for the last eighteen months. The marriage has been badly affected by Dawn's urinary infections, perineal soreness, operations, drugs and general debilitations. Dawn, desperately needing the simple human comfort of being held and reassured, moved back into the double bed last week. They have not had intercourse.

Life-style

In 1976, when all Dawn's trouble seemed to begin, she and Gregory coincidentally moved house. My questioning then tried to establish any link and was minute in detail. The queries involved the old bungalow and the new house.

Bungalow   In its bathroom was a bath, toilet, basin and a hand-shower. Dawn bathed, she did not shower.

New house   In its bathroom there is a bath, toilet, basin and separate shower cubicle. Dawn now showers.

Gregory has had haemorrhoids for many years and has two flannels for his own hygiene which are hung over the side of the handbasin. Dawn says he did the same in the bungalow.

Hygiene

Dawn does not pass a stool regularly and all the antibiotics have increased the constipation, but she doesn't go longer than two days without taking a laxative. She swore that from receiving my books two weeks ago she had got the hygiene right. SHE HAD NOT. Although I've known worse efforts, whatever she was doing either by wrong hand movements or in the soaping, she wasn't absolutely correct. This is how she described the last fortnight's hygiene since receiving my book and it bears little resemblance to my detailed instructions!

- Used toilet paper from the back. *OK.*
- Put any brand of soap on wet cotton wool and wiped perineum, flushed cotton wool away. *Not OK.*
- Reached for a bottle, filled it with warm water and poured it from front to back down the perineum. *OK.*
- Does not use right hand to ensure complete removal of soapy liquid and faecal remnants whilst bottled water is in flow. *Not OK.*
- Reaches for a small towel and dries the perineum from the front. *OK.*

She was rigorously taken through the bottle-washing procedure – twice!

General health

There is no major illness running through her family and she herself has had no other health troubles of the present grim proportions. She feels ill, looks exhausted, white and strained.

Diet, clothing and liquid intake

Were satisfactory and, in any case, are inconsequential.

My suggestions (just as they were written in counselling)

1. Move Gregory's hygiene flannels to separate wall hooks.
2. Dilatations and bladder stretches cause scarring, which becomes weaker skin and more tolerant to bacterial invasions.
3. Lack of hormones also enables skin to accept bacterial invasion.

4   The two separate courses of hormone treatment were insufficient to draw any conclusions.

5   You may need more hormone treatment, possibly continuous OR for at least six months OR until you feel well.

6   Go back to the private gynaecologist who tried the Premarin tablets, show him this list of suggestions and ask whether you may have a six-month course, then analysis and discussion.

7   The scar and labial injury from the old fall will add weakened skin to the irritating, ageing perineal and vaginal skin.

8   The hygiene at any of your stages could have encouraged E. Coli or other bowel bacteria to invade the urethra, especially with the scratching, too.

9   Keep a watch-out for thrush following antibiotics even though you appear never to have it.

10   Antibiotics will also help make you feel run-down, tired and ill.

11   So will lack of hormones.

12   Correct hormone levels mean healthier bladder tissue and urethral skin.

13   Take plenty of vitamins and minerals.

14   Basically I feel it's a combination of:
    (a)   various scar tissues following operations
    (b)   ineffective perineal hygiene and
    (c)   ageing urethral/vaginal skin

My comments

Many of the women who come to me for counselling have 'been everywhere', 'done everything' and are at the end of their tether. Dawn was! She was ill, angry and fearful, and I had to pull her up time and again when the answer to a question or command was not right.

For instance, up in the bathroom when I had sat on the edge of the bath and sat her on the closed toilet lid to describe to me her washing procedure after passing a stool, she did not heed my careful instruction to do exactly that. After supposedly passing a stool (all pretend)! she reached for the loo paper and moved it immediately to wipe from the front. I wrote that hand movement straight on to my notes. On a subsequent hand movement later in the proceedings she moved from the front again and I queried it by saying, 'after a stool?' 'No,' she replied, 'after passing urine.'

I took her right back and made her start all over again because it was obvious that she had not listened at the start. It did transpire that she does wipe with toilet paper from the back and not from the front after passing a stool.

She was also a little muddle-headed from the depressing life which now restricted her, as, for instance, in apologizing for not settling easily into my early conversations with the reasoning that it was 'because of the menopause'. Strictly speaking, you don't have a menopause if you've had a hysterectomy. Ageing does cause lowering hormone levels but she could not have explained it like that.

What sticks in my throat is the urological treatment. A negative kidney X-ray, a negative micturating cystogram, three negative cystoscopies (2 NHS, 1 private) and THEN *two* totally unnecessary urethral dilatations and *three* totally unnecessary bladder stretches! It sounds just like America – that's the sort of treatment cystitis patients get there. Unhappily, there are some general surgeons and urologists who will use these crazy, fashionable treatments left over from the late 1960s and mid-1970s.

They don't work. In only one well-recognized area of female urology is dilatation indicated – that is when a condition called interstitial cystitis has been diagnosed. The bladder is diseased and slowly contracting in size to the point where it just can't function any more. The stretching and dilating every three months help to keep some bladder size and function ability. American women are far more frequently diagnosed as having this condition than their British counterparts. It's rare here, but over 30,000 women in the States are now recipients of this diagnosis.

Ever suspicious, I fear that part of the reason can be found in the private medicine of America, which makes more money from operating than by consultation or self-help. I once knew the medical secretary to a busy gynaecologist in New York who, along with her colleagues in the practice, was told to ask each patient on the phone whether she was bleeding in between periods. If the answer was yes, the secretaries were instructed to move that patient to the next day's list and to telephone the less remunerative patient to make an excuse and a new appointment!

Once you begin on dilatations the urologists seem fond of suggesting more, but each dilatation leaves further inert scar tissue.

Dawn does not have interstitial cystitis. I asked her whether she had ever heard this word and repeated it fully for her to hear. She shook her head and obviously had not had it mentioned to her at any time. If she *does* have interstitial cystitis and doesn't know it because they haven't thought fit to *tell* her in three years, then I suggest she takes it up with her Member of Parliament!

When she said that she'd moved house in 1976 and that seemed to her to be the year when trouble began, I waited with some excitement to hear whether she'd put a bidet in the new bathroom. She hadn't, but it's interesting to look at the bathing and showering. In the bungalow she bathed and had no urinary symptoms; in the new house urinary tract infections began. I wondered whether I could find any sort of reason for this but it would have needed more time. For instance, I would have liked to ask:

- Did you bath at a different *time* of the day from now?
- Did you bath more often then than you shower now?

But a superficial reason, without deep questioning and demonstrating, might be that when you stand upright, as against sitting in the bath, gravity can direct the actual point at which the water drips off your trunk to being slightly *forward* of the dangerous rectal orifice, allowing faecal remnants to move nearer the vagina and urethra. Those women who, until I tell them not to, will squat in the bath and use a handshower, possibly have this gravity influence too.

My own hygiene is primarily:

- Washing with the bottle method after any bowel movement.
- A proper bath twice weekly. I don't like showering, I feel tense about falling over and chilly if I fail to adjust the water easily.

If I was sweaty, which I'm not, I'd wash underarm at the basin with a flannel just like our great grandmothers had to! Actually, come to think of it, I often do wash like that; I did this morning!

Dawn's 'fingering' and 'scratching' of her irritated perineum might also be spreading the unremoved E.Coli, or whatever, towards the urethral orifice. I don't really think that Gregory's very unhygienic placing of his own flannels on the generally used bathroom basin are influencing things. If they are, it's a remote possibility because he's *always* put them there in both houses over some fifteen years or more, Dawn says.

Between the ages of 36 and 43, i.e. from the hysterectomy to the start of symptoms, is a fair number of years, and it could well take that long in a young woman for early symptoms of lowering hormone levels to show up. Certainly from 43 to her current age of 51 we might expect, and actually see, signs of hormone imbalance. The single month's course of Premarin would not be nearly enough to remove the now serious symptoms. An implant might be better for her.

Her life quality is as low as it can get without someone suggesting psychiatric intervention – a favourite step by some doctors in my experience – or just simply retiring to bed for ever!

I could do a fair-size paper on the subject of women and tranquillizers over the age of 45 or after childbirth. I could also quote some of my past patients who have received very distressing electrode treatments for 'imagining your symptoms' and one horrendous twenty-year-long case history ending in lobotomy. A lobotomy is performed on that part of the brain which is involved with pain and tensions.

That particular woman, after being treated by her nearest menopause clinic for severe hormone imbalance some twenty years after a youthful hysterectomy, recovered in three months, rang me to thank me for my help and said that the clinic to which I had referred her stated that they would support her if she wanted to bring any action against her previous doctors for having committed her three times to a mental hospital for many months at a time and finally performing the lobotomy. I don't think she ever did bring an action – she said that she hadn't the time because she now had to pack twenty lost years into her remaining ones! She is still on hormone treatment.

Worse still is, of course, suicide. Again, more women than men commit it. Yet our minds are as strong as theirs, with the exception of the effects on the outlook on life influenced by hormone levels. Why won't doctors stand back from their insistence on categorizing patients into medical niches regardless of the patient's signals and frustrations? What's wrong with applying some old fashioned common sense and a Sherlock Holmes' attitude?

Back to Dawn! We'll have to give her 2–3 months for any

prescribed hormone treatment to become beneficial and, hopefully, now urinary infection will be a thing of the past with new, more effective hygiene and healthier skin.

Again, I wish I felt that I could trust the doctors into whose care I am forced to return her. Despite my ideas, there could well be other factors that my super gynaecologists might discover on examination and which would influence the case.

Just as Dawn was walking out through the front door, she asked my opinion on how she should manage the school board assessment meetings next week. With three months being a reasonable time for any resulting benefits from the hormones and hygiene to be seen, I suggested that she might ask the board for a stay of decision until Christmas and, naturally, she would have to explain why.

If, unhappily, my current ideas do not resolve the symptoms, then I suggested that she does come to London for further gynaecological investigations. But by then the school board may well have run out of patience and reluctantly pension her off.

Follow-up – November

Dawn rang me for support and information. Her GP totally agreed with my suggestions after she had reported back to him. The comments on the scarring caused by those seemingly unnecessary urological operations were supported, though I am forced to query his ready acceptance of such drastic work when the specialists wrote to him. Why hadn't he advised her against them then?

The soreness and urinary involvement have continued, but recent urine tests have stopped showing E.Coli. Dawn's new washing is having a beneficial effect.

The GP is now fully committed to getting her hormone levels right and again is in full agreement with me. An early appointment was kept with the best gynaecologist in the area, but it resulted in a different administration than we had hoped for. He has put her on a very low-dose hormone tablet for two years and has said that he doesn't want to see her again for twelve months. This low dosage takes account of the adverse reaction which she experienced on a high-dose tablet last year. The GP and I believe that she needs an implant and Dawn rang me for a discussion of what her GP had said. I gave my opinion:

1   Continue on the low dose tablet and give it much more time.

2   Connive with the GP to find another gynaecologist locally who would do an implant.

3   Come down to London for a consultation with the specialist to whom I refer women with severe hormone imbalance and who uses implanted hormones very successfully.

I feel that the treatment is not in question, only the most effective way of implementing it.

Follow-up – January

Dawn, out of the occasional bouts of impatience when painful symptoms flare up, in frustration turns back to a urologist. At such times she is her own worst enemy. Three recent days of bladder pain, not pain on passing urine but an internal pain which she describes as 'bladder' pain, sent her flying off to another urologist, who has put her on Urispas tablets for two months and then suggested another bladder stretch if the Urispas doesn't work. I made her promise not to let that happen!

We talked the bladder pain through:

- It's not there all the time.
- Sometimes she's without it for many days.
- The urine doesn't sting or burn.
- Those awful bladder scars will react to many outside factors such as very cold weather or temporary insufficient liquid in the bladder.
- With one ovary left there may still be evidence of cycles affecting hormonal activity. Her bladder may be responding to this.
- I've asked her to ring me when she panics and feels like rushing off for more urological intervention. She's only done it the once.
- No infections for two months.
- Why hasn't she been to see the hormone specialist in London?

The answer to the last question was money and the bad weather. Well, moneywise, she's spending it on private consultations anyway! All past urological treatment has failed to come up with an answer and the costly investigations have found nothing wrong at all. As for the weather, the trains still run and main streets are reasonably clear of snow.

The real reason, I suspect, is that she is inclined to focus on the bladder as a *cause* and not a *result* of another cause, e.g. the hormone deficiency.

I asked her to list anything beneficial resulting from these mild but slow-acting hormone tablets that she has now taken for four months.

1 The major symptoms of soreness and perineal irritation which she listed in October as the number one problem have all but disappeared, recurring now only sporadically.
2 The backache, again a big symptoms, has almost gone, only recurring occasionally and then not badly.
3 She feels brighter, not so depressed.
4 She now only gets up twice a night to pass urine, not every hour.

These are major improvements, but because they are happening extremely slowly Dawn is almost unaware of them except when pressed to concentrate on them. There may even be other improvements which she doesn't know about, like healthier internal skin.

These improvements have taken four months; who knows what another four months will bring? It's hard for her to wait, but the bladder has taken a hell of a pounding from medical intervention over the years and has, at the same time, been struggling on, like the vagina and perineum, with lowering hormone levels.

Dawn, I am still convinced, is driving to the right destination. It's just that perhaps by not having an implant, she has taken the old route through the centre of a congested town instead of driving swiftly round the modern bypass!

Dramatically, but not unexpectedly, she has lost her job with the meals service of the local education authority. She has been pensioned off by the council with a very small monthly sum, and Dawn and her husband have estimated that she has lost £64,000 of remaining salary between now and normal retirement age.

A very recent phone call has revealed that she is not getting up at all now in the night, that she is brighter and able to do a full load of ironing in one session. The bladder pain is no longer a pain but more of a tingle and irritation, and this is probably happening every three weeks lasting for five to six days. The remaining ovary may still be running on a cycle and accounting for this pattern. Dawn is going to keep a diary for two months.

When I rang, I didn't recognize her voice: it was lighter and brighter. I asked if I could speak to Mrs Carling, and when she replied that it was her, I knew instantly that she was improving tremendously!

All those urological operations failed, yet two simple hormone tablets taken daily now for five full months have worked wonders. I ,suggested she get information from the Ombudsman and a special solicitor to see whether through the courts she can recover at least some money to compensate for the ineffective handling of her suffering and loss of salary both past and future. I don't think she will, though. She's not that sort of a person.

CHAPTER NINE

Mrs Brenda Lincoln

Brenda Lincoln, aged 51, lives with her husband Barry in Cheshire. She is now chronically disabled with multiple sclerosis and was, from her phone call to me, obviously unable to travel to London, so I visited her. Barry met me at the station and in fifteen minutes we were drawing up under cover beside the wheelchair ramp at their front door. The house is a very pleasant modern bungalow, which Barry has adapted to suit Brenda's needs. He has removed two of the three bedrooms and built on a den all by himself. The main bedroom now has a large and beautifully designed bathroom area, which used to be one of the other bedrooms. A lot of money has been spent on sanitary equipment to help life along, and it all looked terrific – not the least bit medical.

Barry is jolly and, despite disc trouble last year, is playing the part of supporter and husband as well as anyone could. He likes football and used to garden but doesn't anymore. He works in the offices of a nearby nuclear power station.

Brenda, once she had graduated, went to work with ICI until advanced multiple sclerosis finally forced her to take early retirement in 1981. She does as much of her own housework as she can manage and she reads a bit, but mostly by lunchtime her energies are flagging. She says that she doesn't feel ill as illness goes, but obviously you can't be classified well if you spend your days in a wheelchair!

She has been in the wheelchair since 1972, but until January 1984, when she broke her right leg, she was able to stand and take the odd step. Prior to 1972 she managed well enough on sticks.

She sits dead square and upright in the hated wheelchair and, although she is probably a slim to middlish size 16, she fills the not over-generous dimensions of the National Health Service chair. Because her shoulders aren't supported and because of the MS, she slumps slowly and periodically replaces herself upright once more. Her dark hair is close-cropped and she wears no make-up; her knee-length dress is of royal blue patterned Thai cotton, lined with a polyester mix.

Today, she tells me, she is not wearing her cotton knickers because this particular dress does have a skirt lining. The plastic seat of the NHS wheelchair is usually covered with a folded towel upon which she sits.

Barry provided some delicious tea and gooey cakes from the bakery then departed, and Brenda and I sat at the sunny dining table to begin.

Symptoms

A non-irritant, slightly pinkish vaginal discharge, which Brenda thinks is thrush. It can be streaky. It has been present ever since she went in the wheelchair in 1972. There has never been any urinary trouble, ever. There is no backache, pelvic ache, pain or irritation. MS sufferers apparently get migrainous neuralgia – nasty headaches – but special drugs are prescribed for this and she now seldom gets a headache.

The great void in a reliable diagnosis of this thrush is that she has never been examined for it – never! Neither by the somewhat difficult local medical staff nor by her neurologist nor by any gynaecologist. No swabs have ever been taken in the twelve years in which she has had it. Her GP has taken her word for it being thrush and has prescribed Nizoral and Nystatin pessaries.

Gynaecological history

Periods began at 14 and were normal. She has never had any kind of gynaecological examination or operation, and I had to describe to her the very basics of examination from lying down on the couch.

Children

None, and has never been pregnant.

Sex

Until thrush began in 1972 she and Barry obviously enjoyed inter-course. From 1972 it became rather sporadic, several times a month instead of several times a week. This continued until January 1984 when she broke her leg and was encased in plaster, after having to insist on an X-ray to prove the break. A week of great pain had ensued before the doctors were agreeable to this X-ray. So sex went by the wayside, what with the plaster and resulting tenderness. By June it had still not be resumed.

Menopause

Make of this what you will, but Brenda's periods stopped in 1979 whilst in the Manchester Royal Infirmary for a course of hydro-therapy and physiotherapy. Having arrived, the hydrotherapy pool promptly went out of action because of a strike by engineers and she waited on in the hope that it would be all right 'the next day'. In six weeks the pool was opened for use twice and each time Brenda was put in it. Whilst home for a weekend she called the GP complaining of feeling sick and feverish. The GP referred her back to the infirmary, where she was returning the next day anyway! Streptococci were found from a urine sample and she was given antibiotics. Two weeks later a nasty pus-filled leg ulcer developed, culturing the same strain of streptococci. The pool was blamed. Further antiobiotics and leg dressings were administered and the ulcer cleared completely. She has not needed antibiotics since then for anything. Her periods stopped in those six weeks and have not returned.

General

She is given injections and steroids and is not on cortisone. Vitamin B12 is an added supplement. A senior physiotherapist comes twice weekly to give bed exercises but Brenda has lost confidence in the ability of the leg to hold her up. Because of Barry's disc and back trouble their bed was changed for a firmer one, but this has different dimensions and Brenda cannot get herself on to it unaided. Barry helps her on and off it, but naturally this only happens around 10.30 at night and 7.30 in the morning. Thus Brenda says there is no time to do the necessary leg exercises. She sits with the perineum pressured from the wheelchair and is prevented by the dimensions of the wheelchair from shifting this pressure because the wheelchair's sides and back are narrow and rigid. She can't part her thighs to let air reach the perineum.

Clothing

Disabled patients adapt ordinary clothing to facilitate ease of dressing. Jeans, skirts and flesh-hugging undies can't be worn. Brenda wears loose-fitting cotton knickers, Polly Peck 'hold-ups', nylon/polyester petticoats and dresses. Because of the leg plaster it was not even possible to get knickers on, so she took to putting the towel on the wheelchair seat.

She admits to getting overwarm at night in bed. Her nighties are polyester/cotton and she has the same mixture for her sheets. The duvet is down-filled and she was thinking of changing it for a lighter one filled with terylene, but I recommended blankets instead.

Food and liquid

Brenda is not overweight for her age and height. She has one teaspoonful of sugar in coffee twice a day and sugar on cereals in the morning. Every day she has a large glass of lemonade and will have a couple of glasses of red wine about twice a month when they got out for a meal.

Hygiene

Brenda showers once a week in the special shower that Barry has installed. In between, they use a remarkable lavatory called a Clos-O-Mat which had been originally designed to help a severely tortured British ex-prisoner of war from Japan (so they told me).

This lavatory has two elbow-pressure controls, one for flushing and the other for starting a shower action down in the bowl. The small showerhead can be extended and angled so that its spray reaches further forward on the perineum, but will not flow from front to back. I tried this thing on a last-minute impulse, and its action is from back to front – highly dangerous for women. The showerhead is sited centre left of the back of the lavatory bowl – fine, I suppose, for men (remember, it was designed for one) but dreadful for women. All her faecal material is propelled forward.

It's frankly amazing that Brenda doesn't have continuous urinary infections. I was also told that it is widely used in maternity homes, and I must investigate this some day.

My suggestions

1 Insist on a good vaginal examination. This non-irritative pinkish discharge, although stringy, does not have true thrush symptoms. It could be anything.

2 Use the VD/genito-urinary clinic at Manchester, thus by passing the tetchy local medical staff who, by now, should have investigated the discharge anyway. The VD unit uses instant microscope analysis (something which Brenda appreciated) and will give immediate appropriate treatment.

3 This discharge could be from cervical erosion or polypus.

4 Remember to go for a clearance swab after any treatment.

5 Thrush breeds in warmth and moisture (conditions much aided by sitting in the wheelchair), so to try and get round this:

   (a) When Barry returns home from work around 6 p.m., go on the bed. This will enable the leg exercises to be done and air to get to the perineum. Pressure is off the perineum, too. It's a three-fold benefit.

   (b) Try wearing long, full cotton caftans so that you present a more elegant frontage to the world whilst bed exercising!

   (c) When the exercises have sufficiently strengthened the leg to enable it to take some weight, you will be able to stand a little and remove the perineal pressure, whilst aiding air access.

   (d) Go without pants as often as possible.

   (e) In winter, wear long woollen vests and warm caftans but keep the perineum clear for air access.

6 Cut out all sugar, since thrush – if it *is* thrush – loves sugar.

7 Even that small alcohol intake can upset the sugar balance, if it is thrush.

8 How about a cool hot-water bottle at night to reduce heat in bed?

9 Find bedding that is easy-care but less warm.

10 Cut pubic hair to ½ inch in length. Brenda can't manage to

use scissors and wouldn't ask Barry, but the district nurse, not currently visiting, ought to do so every 6–8 weeks.

11 Try requesting Gynodaktarin anti-fungal cream and Nystatin oral tablets if tests show the discharge to be thrush.

12 Use the bottle process for washing. A hard thing to say in view of Barry's wonderful bathroom, but I remain very suspicious of the Clos-O-Mat. Brenda may find a glass bottle too difficult to hold, in which case a plastic bottle with handle might be found. This portable washing process might enable her to visit hotels where washing facilities are not so helpful.

13 A final thought – how are the hormones doing since the complete cessation of periods?

My comments

Both Brenda and Barry are survivors. They survive with attention to daily detail, with lively minds, with a cheering, well-run home and with a lot of cherishing of one another. It is not possible to speak too highly of a man at work who comes home and supports his wife in her trouble, nor of her whose gentle and practical responses to being helped are so ungrudgingly given.

That being said, my knowledge and help on thrush was, I felt, somewhat thwarted because Brenda could not give even one absolute medical confirmation that she has thrush. I wouldn't be prepared to put money on it and hope very much to know what the VD/genito-urinary clinic makes of the discharge. The description 'pinkish' was not even reminiscent of ordinary daily vaginal mucous, and I really needed to have taken a doctor with me.

It is quite awful that, even though they live a little way out of a big city – some 15 miles from Manchester – in a small town, their medical help is so unsupportive. Why didn't her local GP suggest that he examine her when she first asked for treatment for thrush? Why should she have to feel the need to ring me a couple of hundred miles away? I am glad that she did, of course, and hope the suggestions will give her something to work on.

Follow-up – August

On the telephone it was perfectly obvious that Mrs Lincoln had been crying. Her nose sounded blocked and she didn't mention having a cold. Very shortly, the reason became clear. Three weeks ago she strained her back and has been given a three-and-a-half-month recovery period from a severely pulled muscle. She is on heavy doses of a strong painkiller, which is causing acute constipation – a great difficulty when confined to a wheelchair and in pain.

There is still no health visitor or practitioner visiting. The physiotherapist is coming once a week, although he cannot work on the leg because of the severe back pain. I suggested that a letter to the local medical staff requesting that a vaginal swab be taken at home might be written and Brenda may do this; but she has little faith left in the caring of these locals and, because there is no other health centre near her, she feels that she must save her requirements and requests only for dire emergencies.

This is a truly disgraceful state of affairs. It highlights in great intensity the chasm between a five-figure sum spent on a chancy heart-swap operation and spending a minimal amount on a humdrum life-quality situation.

My interest in Brenda is only connected with one small part of her suffering – i.e. a simple vaginal swab to find out what her discharge contains and treat it if necessary – but short of marching up to her front door with a gynaecologist in tow, I am about as much help to her as petrol is to a car without wheels. I found this a depressing case and remain very grateful for my own blessings.

CHAPTER TEN

Mrs Sonia Moreille

This lady is 50. She doesn't look a day over 40, and a gynaecologist actually said recently that her skin, muscle tone and general health is that of a woman ten years younger.

When she approached me after a lecture to a business women's group and gave me the briefest of descriptions amounting to possible prolapse of the uterus making her slightly incontinent, I asked her to come for counselling. (Stress urgency of urination is a common problem, and I feel that the book has a place for such a history.)

At that moment I remember saying that I normally mention surgery of any sort as the last resort and never suggest it casually. But here was a young woman in her late thirties (I thought) with two children (young ones, I thought) and repairing a prolapse now might prevent it enlarging. A sort of stitch-in-time-saves-nine situation.

Sonia, in counselling, turned out to be fifty. Impossible to believe! She arrived without make-up – apparently unusual for her since she puts it on when travelling on the underground – and her dark brown hair fringed across her forehead and dropped straight down to her shoulders. Within this brown frame a finely honed bone structure was softened by two big brown eyes showing much intelligence and directness. Sonia wore a beautiful brown wool superbly tailored culotte suit, sheer dark brown stockings and real lizardskin walking shoes. Pricey but tasteful.

She is an artist. She also has a degree in science but doesn't use it. On arrival in England from Australia she worked as an art teacher in London, but has stopped that this year. Occasionally she writes poetry and used to run a workshop but has now confined her poems to the attic. Two children, both attending a day school in London, form her immediate family, but her mother is also still alive and living in England despite being given three months to live in 1957 because of cancer!

This year has seen the latest chapter of her passionately tempestuous love affair with an almost mentally unstable but brilliant architect in Australia. They parted in August, yet again, with many acrimonious insults flung from trains, planes and reams of notepaper.

Sonia is still under Harry's spell after 14 years, and since removing herself from him in August is only a shadow of herself. Not an hour goes by without her referring to him in her thoughts. Most of our counselling was directly associated with him because his behaviour causes her much emotional upset, and this affects the severity of her particular stress urgency. So to exclude him would have discouraged a useful dialogue between us on her urinary symptoms.

Richard and Nell, her two teenage children, are from her only marriage, which lasted from 1958 to 1979. The divorce took a full eight years and was difficult. It is mostly because of them that Sonia and Harry argue; Harry wants her to be totally dependent on him and with him twenty-four hours a day – one step away from being chained up. They have long breaks, for which he has taken time off work, so that sex can become their only occupation. Five or six times a day for many days at a time are a delight, a fantasy and an impossible way to carry on if you have two children, let alone children from a former marriage. Sonia and Harry alternately passionately rape each other and row with each other. The rows are the reverse swing of the pendulum and it is usually during these swings that the urinary symptoms become embarrassingly troublesome.

Over the years she has, in love and duty, cared for her children and seen to their schooling in England. Long spells in Nepal, Egypt, Canada and Australia make for a globe-trotting bent enhanced by a consuming lust for Harry's body. As Sonia says, this is the stuff of fantasy, and there must be many women who would happily fantasize in such thoughts but not actually want to live with the nightmarish results of such fantasy brought to life. Most would say 'it's not worth it'. Sonia would say that she's trapped, does her best to throw Harry off and work at her family duties, but descends into gloom and despair when he is not there and she is not having intercourse. She does not sleep around, despite many men finding her earthily attractive.

Since the August row, she and Harry have communicated in only three letters. His second letter told her that he wished she were dead, and because she'd gone away he was marrying someone else very soon. Sonia hasn't replied and is extremely bitter that his often irrational demands are too much when other parts of life just have to be lived too. She can't stay in bed all year at his disposal, even though she'd love to.

This latest and lengthy separation has reduced her morale and her mental and physical well being to a very low level. She is doing nothing except housework and childcare. Her artistic talents are lying fallow and broken, her femininity is zero and she wants Harry badly, even through the bitterness. At least she is doing some gym work-outs, keeping a good vitamin intake and trying to improve on the physical difficulties. The depression from having no sex and no Harry is making her lethargic and giving rise to minor stress-induced ailments. She is into reflexology for liver malfunction and into electro-pulsed magnetic therapy.

Reflexology is the action of pressure on points in the feet and other limbs which will stimulate specific organs elsewhere into a stronger performance.

Electro-pulsed magnetic therapy is useful for faster healing of injured bones or muscular injuries. It can also help repel infections and inflammations. The Queen, other members of the Royal Family, jockeys, skiers and many women with poor pelvic health are just some of the people who can benefit from electro-pulsed magnetic therapy. Sonia feels stronger from this treatment to her uterus. She feels that the stress incontinence is lessening but no one, naturally, is going to prove that.

Symptoms

Frequency and stress incontinence. There were many urinary infections before marriage in 1958 but none since. At times the incontinence will cause urine to flood down her legs if a lavatory is not quickly available; on some occasions Sonia will rise from a chair with wet pants; and at other times, like sneezing or walking fast, urine will splash or jerk out of the urethral tube. Whenever she is near a lavatory she will use it, but even so, the wetness seldom stops. The emotional situation since the recent walk-out has seen the incontinence worsen with the stress. Without intercourse, the vaginal epithelium (skin) will become unhealthy and clogged up with heavy white mucous.

Urological history

Before marriage, MSUs always showed bacteria – but none since.
IVP: None
Last saw a urologist in 1962
Cystoscopy 1960, without anaesthetic. She still remembers the pain.

Gynaecological history

Periods began when she was 13 and were so awful that Sonia took to her bed for three days each month vomiting and flooding. In Australia when she was 34, a gynaecologist started her on injections of Depoprovera – a progesterone (male) based hormone. After all the past years of trying many treatments, including various oestrogen (female) therapies, this injection completely stopped the periods and helped the premenstrual tension, whilst also becoming her contraceptive. Her breasts became breasts and she took on a healthy weight of nine and a half stone.

In 1984 a British gynaecologist decided to stop the Depoprovera, with Sonia's agreement (and her weight has resumed its earlier eight stone, periods are back but behaving reasonably. When the first injection after stopping became due, she felt ill. Vaginal health has become poor, breasts are tiny and she is greatly depressed. This was compounded by the row and walk-out, which unhappily coincided within a few weeks.

In September 1984 a gynaecological examination showed prolapse of the uterus. This prolapse does not descend yet into the cervix and vagina, so the gynaecologist did not classify an operation to stitch it up as urgent. He did suggest that she thinks about having surgery.

A displaced uterus pressurizes the bladder lying close next door, and it will work involuntarily – hence Sonia's particular kind of urgency and frequency.

Contraceptives

None needed currently but the Depoprovera acted for this purpose.

Babies

One boy, 1967. Vaginal delivery, severely torn and heavily stitched. One girl, 1969. Vaginal delivery, marvellous and only minor stitching.

Sex

None currently for six months. Otherwise sporadic, according to state of relationship with Harry. When this is good, sex is almost continuous sometimes for weeks at a time. Totally enthralling and pain-free, with Harry, at 59 now, still very virile. He used to treat her with some force and the subjugation only added to the sexual intensities, making her really forever reliant on him.

General

Sonia visits a gym and sauna every Sunday for four and a half hours. She takes Vitamin E, which is an antioxidant, and garlic capsules for stress. The Alexander technique for body and posture awareness, together with reflexology, is practised once a week with a therapist – Vida Menzies, of 127 Ebury Street, London SW1. The electro-pulsed magnetic therapy and massage are practised by Kay Kiernan and her staff, of 16 Harley House, Marylebone Road, London NW1. Out of all this, Sonia is striving to overcome her problems and keep mentally afloat. She feels that the reflexology has perhaps eased the wetness but has not yet stopped it.

My suggestions and comments

I felt that I might be helpful in two ways.

First, I dealt with the wetness and incontinence. Although Sonia feels this has improved, it hasn't stopped. I put it to her that, as she was doing so much to try to help herself, had she thought of seeing to the prolapse also? It seems a shame not to pay attention to this when so much else is being done along other lines of work. So I gave the name of a gynaecologist in lieu of the one who had first reported the prolapse but then moved hospitals. Prolapses tend to worsen, and so even though the uterus hasn't yet descended down the cervical canal, a stitch in time could well save nine, as I had first commented after meeting Sonia at the lecture.

Second, far from what her friends are saying about the tempestuous affair with Harry and recommending to Sonia that she abandon him to what he deserves, including the threatened marriage, I offered a different idea. This affair of 14 years has to be counted as a very real relationship. Not a common one, granted, but nonetheless it is the one which has featured in Sonia's life. She is obviously bereft without him but equally obviously cannot possibly submit to his demands of leaving her children and lying underneath him at all hours in Australia!

That being recognized, I suggested she thinks about writing to him upon his marriage – which is probably being undertaken, if at all, out of revenge and acidness – and hope that they might meet up on any architectural conferences, symposiums etc. These are planned well in advance at different locations around the world, far away from placing any hurt on his marriage.

Sonia loved this! Morals and ethics apart, it was the first recognition by anyone that she had a gut need of Harry. Everyone else is telling her to live on without him. After six months, she's hardly managing to, and the hope that I seemed to generate has probably done more good than all the garlic capsules ever manufactured.

A lot of modern life is lived out in this secretive fashion, and if one man keeps two distant women in good health it actually could be regarded as a medical service. Women have for centuries been saying that men are only good for one thing. Well, let it be so! The man living who has not once committed adultery is singularly rare. Adultery is still a marriage wrecker, and will be in the future; but we don't live in villages any more, nor do women always conceive a child from it – thanks to contraceptives. A lot of the ancient reasons for not committing adultery are no longer here.

Some sort of regular sex life is essential for female health. The vagina stays in tone, monthly tensions and general mental health are improved. Sex is far preferable to sleeping pills, tranquillizers, and drink and drug abuse. Any good doctor will tell you this. If divorce is becoming a sad acceptance in today's world, then the same reluctant acceptance of adultery, quietly done, must follow. We must arrive back at the social acknowledgement of mistresses, once commonplace and now out of fashion for a century.

Follow-up – February

Sonia has done nothing that I suggested! That is to say, she hasn't needed to. She cannot directly point to which of the two treatments was responsible because she was undergoing both of them at the same time. As she says, it's hard to be systematic about choosing one treatment and sticking with it for some months by itself when you're totally fed up with being incapacitated. If you've several options, it's tempting to try more than one at a time and not wait. This is what has happened to her.

For several weeks now, the improvement that she reported to me during our counselling reached a point at Christmas when she suddenly became aware that for two days she had been absolutely dry. There were no gushes of urine down her legs nor had she had to rush for a lavatory.

This happy state of regained continence remained and is still there, even a fair amount of walking around Paris on a weekend visit failed to cause one anxious moment, and she felt that to be an excellent test.

So how has this come about and would anyone be likely to explain it scientifically?

Reflexology and electro-pulsed magnetic therapy are new concepts to the majority of the lay and medical population. They were unknown in England fifteen years ago and doubtless have more sceptics than devotees. But, ever true to my own philosophy – which is: never make rock-hard rules for patients – I concede that Sonia, as a result of either of the treatments, is now well. She wasn't well BEFORE them but she *is* well AFTER them – you can't just sniff at an intelligent woman and reject what she says out of hand. You must ask nice questions out of curiosity and a wish to understand better. The treatments may only work for some people and not others; who knows?

Unless Sonia were to submit to conventional gynaecological re-appraisal of her reported prolapse, it would be impossible to judge whether the prolapse, has miraculously vanished; or whether the surrounding muscles and ligaments have been sufficiently improved to compensate and restrain the bladder functions regardless of the prolapsed section. Therefore we must conclude that we cannot, as yet, account for the disappearance of her incontinence.

The pressures that Vida Menzies applied to a toe on Sonia's right foot (it can be either foot), the underneath of the instep and just below the ankle bones, again on the right foot, were sometimes so acute that Sonia screamed and asked her to stop. Vida Menzies replied that it was doing a lot of good to the bladder, and kept on!

Kay Kiernan and her staff have been blasting positive ions into Sonia's pelvic region and her adrenals to improve the blood supply at the same time as the reflexology treatment. The ions are invisible and soundless, coming out of a little black box plugged into the mains electricity. A metal disc positioned on any part of the body is aided by a flexible metal arm – like one of those adjustable desk-lamps. The patient lies down fully dressed, covered in blankets, and relaxes whilst the positioned disc gets to work. Exposure to the ions usually lasts an hour, no longer. You don't feel anything at all during the treatment.

Sonia has been diligently taking the black-box treatment for about four months now and will shortly go on once-monthly maintenance therapy.

I asked her whether the reflexologist thinks that the incontinence has gone for ever, and Vida Menzies has implied that she thinks it has; but, of course, only time will really tell.

This is quite marvellous for Sonia. Whatever makes you well is absolutely right for you, and don't let anyone make you feel stupid or insignificant when you explain what *has* made you well. If they laugh, laugh back – it's your body that's feeling better, not theirs, and you shouldn't give a damn what they think!

As for the sex life, Sonia apparently has 'opportunities' but prefers to bide her time until the right man comes along. She's not promiscuous and she does have a family to consider. She also still loves Harry, and the memories are inclined to slip back into her mind.

After thinking through what I had suggested, she felt that Harry would still be controlling their affair, since she would be largely dependent upon his dates for meeting, not hers, so she's still struggling hard to reconcile herself and her bodily needs to living without him. She hasn't written to him nor has she received any communication from him, but a girlfriend in Australia is keeping a weather eye out!

Those of you with incontinence due to minor or suspected prolapse might like to note this history because, if you've tried most things to gain relief, perhaps you'd like to think about reflexology and/or electro-pulsed magnetic therapy. The latter is claimable on private health insurance, but I'm not sure about reflexology – you'd have to enquire from your health insurance company. Never be afraid to ask a therapist's charges: they would expect you to want to know.

All in all I found this case very interesting, even though I personally did nothing at all. But I learnt a lot instead.

CHAPTER ELEVEN

Mrs Jean Lemmon and Jim

Mrs Lemmon married her husband Jim in 1968 when she was 20. She is now 35 and Jim 41. Their five children range from one to 14 years old and were born between 1970 and 1983. They all live in a large semi-detached house in Harlow New Town, Essex, where regular churchgoing and choir singing provide a base and a rock upon which their family life is lived.

Their hardships have been many, they say, but with a great deal of patience, prayer and persistence and the help of God they are still making it through.

Jim is with a firm making air-conditioning and spends his spare hours as a husband and father. He brought his wife by car to see me, dropped her off whilst he saw a customer and then returned, sitting in on the closing stages of the counselling.

Jean, in between being the fullest of full-time mothers, is doing Advanced Level work on Religious Studies. She clearly states that she and Jim and the last two children are only there because of God and her prayers. They are not Catholics.

She sat down in the armchair rather carefully and collapsed back rather than leant back. She had a pretty spring outfit on with sandals and her hair was tidy, but she still conveyed the feeling of heavy tiredness. A sweet person, this, patient and probably long-suffering. Let's see.

Symptoms

Vaginal soreness. Recent swabs show no thrush. There is apparently a fairly heavy discharge, but the swabs show no abnormal or invasive bacteria. This soreness extends outwards and along the perineum. Twice a year maybe, Jean gets a full-blown attack of cystitis and has come today because cystitis occurred three weeks ago and has not really gone. This latest attack was treated with tablets of Amoxil 500 for seven days. She had cystitis first of all on her honeymoon and periodically ever since.

She has not had cystitis in any one of her five pregnancies, nor when she was on the Pill for a time.

She and Jim had had intercourse 48 hours before this attack and she was very sore afterwards. Since this sequence of events has happened before, her GP has suggested Amoxil might be taken for two days after intercourse. It obviously hasn't worked.

Mostly, though, it's the vaginal soreness which is bothering her. Cystitis twice a year, although bad enough, is not top of her symptoms.

Urological history

Mid-stream urine specimens: usually negative. Occasionally, an unknown something or other is shown.
Intravenous pyelogram: None to date.
Cystoscopy: None.
On 19 June she is to visit another urologist.

Gynaecological history

Periods began aged 13 and were never heavy. There was a lot of pre-menstrual tension. When Jean was 8, she was raped by her brother once and was quite unable to tell anyone, but Jim has been a great comforter. He has been able to talk to her about it so that she has adjusted and settled herself to the memory without needing to seek professional help.

They had a dreadful honeymoon marred by cystitis, the rape memory and tension. On returning home they moved house frequently and spent some time living with in-laws.

Sex

Sporadic and lasts 30 to 40 minutes. Jean isn't sure whether she lubricates sufficiently. Jim is not circumcised, but penetration is smooth and easy enough and Jean feels no lumpy parts or painful ridges whilst intercourse is happening. Sex is more comfortable now but was very uncomfortable after the early babies.

Contraception

The sheath mostly, although there was a spell on the Pill – but Jim and she separated for a short time and she came off it. When he moved back home again she immediately became pregnant and then went on to have two further children, so the sheath was adopted.

Babies

One boy, 1970. Perineal delivery, breast abcess, 18 months of anti-depressants.

One boy, 1973. Another perineal delivery – dreadful and many stitches.

One boy, 1978. Vaginal delivery but sewn so tightly that she needed to return to hospital for stretching. No anaesthetic was given.

One girl, 1980. Vaginal delivery.

One girl, 1983. Vaginal delivery.

Throughout both girl pregnancies, Jean was an exhausted zombie and has remained so a full year after the last baby.

General health

Very tired – the GP says that it isn't surprising, which may or may not be true.

Self-help

Hardly relevant but:

Hygiene

Poor. Washes only with a flannel or cloth and soaps the entire perineum – vaginal and urethra openings included.

Sex

Doesn't use KY Jelly and doesn't wash afterwards.

Food and liquid intake

Doesn't drink alcohol and probably doesn't eat as nourishing meals as her body requires, given its high energy output. Probably doesn't get nearly enough rest.

My suggestions

1 Ask for and receive ALL urine results!
2 Intercourse difficulties over the years have divided into:
  (a) early marriage, trauma and tension
  (b) from 1970, physical trauma with vaginal difficulties caused by birth injuries.
3 Hormones??? That tiredness is not all due to expended energy, I suspect. It coincides too closely with the births and she was once treated (probably wrongly) with anti-depressants. Perhaps the hormone levels are too low.
4 Before intercourse use dollops of KY Jelly to provide extra padding for the vagina and good initial lubrication.
5 The hygiene is poor. Don't use a flannel and never soap the entire perineum.
6 Wash as per the bottle process (demonstrated upstairs) and, with your finger, hook out as much of the vaginal discharge as you can. This will certainly help to keep it off the perineal skin and ease the external soreness.
7 I showed Jean an old-fashioned douche and instructed her about using it correctly. I also showed her a bottle of non-prescribable Betadine Solution whose strength can be diluted to suit each patient. John Bell & Croydon, of Wigmore Street, London W1, would stock this douche, so would many other chemists – but you may have to search a bit. The Betadine Solution can be bought anywhere, but as with any medication, don't use it unless you know what your condition is. Betadine, for instance won't help thrush. Jean's discharge, though heavy, is not apparently showing any bacteria and so the medical profession have pretty well left her to find her own solution.
8 I gave the name of a gynaecologist for assessment of:
  (a) hormone levels
  (b) childbirth injuries
  (c) anything else likely to be causing vaginal soreness and discharge.
9 I suggested that she might think about a two-month experiment on a mini Pill since side-effects before had been negligible and the family is now complete.
10 To help the tiredness levels I suggested long courses of

multivitamins and multiminerals, e.g. Larkhall (Cantassium) Laboratories' 'Zinc and Minerals' tablets.

11 Join a health-insurance company to help with any future medical bills.

My comments

Instinct told me that all here was going to hinge on what the gynaecologist found. My only real self-help advice was to restrain and confine the discharge as much as possible in order not to contaminate the perineal skin. Even the Betadine might be too strong if she really is as sensitive as she says.

Women do sometimes require extra help with minerals and vitamins; here, certainly, is such a time, and I am surprised that the GP has not made some effort in this way.

Jean shouldn't really have waited to be told about the need for belonging to a health-insurance group. The minute you think any illness recently discussed is likely to be a lengthy job, stop work on it and take out some insurance. Wait a bit, see a different doctor if you would like, or return to the first one and go on in the knowledge that you now have some extra monetary help.

Follow-up – July

Jean reported:
- taking the vitamins and minerals regularly
- going on a mini Pill
- washing properly (this is extremely effective and three other people have benefited from her imparted new knowledge, all completely comfortable and praising the bottle method after years of GP ineffectiveness!)
- keeping her previous appointment with the local urologist, which resulted in a negative IVP and much vagueness
- seeing my recommended gynaecologist
- approaching two health-insurance companies for brochures

The gynaecologist's examination and discussion were very fruitful and, as Jean said, a real change from the austere atmosphere in an NHS environment. Pelvic and vaginal muscles are in excellent shape despite the birth horrors, but he found a very heavy vaginal discharge coming off a large area of cervical erosion. This erosion fully accounted for the vaginal soreness which was her prime symptom on her visit to me. Jean says that no NHS examination had reported this erosion. Other investigations which he wants to pursue are fluid-balance charts, which she is now doing at home to help determine whether her intake and output of urine match; cytotoxic tests for body-mineral levels; hormone and thyroid profiles, reference her tiredness.

Jean wrote off to two medical insurances firms: BUPA and WPA.

BUPA will not pay for any treatment of Jean's cystitis since she had it before wanting to join. I did point out that she is not strictly a cystitis patient. Cystitis or urethral twingeing is occurring *as a result* of gynaecological disorders. It is these that need investigation and treatments.

WPA have better preconditions and will accept bills immediately, so Jean is going ahead and registering with them.

Her next appointment with the gynaecologist is on 17 August. The WPA enrolment will by then have been finalized, and investigations and any treatment can commence. Probably, a short general anaesthetic will be given so that the uterus can be fully examined. Whilst she is under, cryo-surgery will be used on the cervical erosion and anywhere else that this erosion has attacked. Other tests don't need an anaesthetic, but one would expect them all to be done in the clinic on that day.

The Betadine Solution proved too strong even when substantially diluted, so Jean stopped using it after only two days. On the other hand, she did report a definite, albeit temporary, easing of the soreness. In view of the gynaecologist's findings, this makes sense. Only when the erosion is removed will the soreness and discharge go for good.

Follow-up – September

Jean's soreness, three weeks after the gynaecologist used cryo-surgery to remove the heavy, infected vaginal/cervical erosion which had also invaded the uterus, is easing considerably. Her intermittent light bouts of soreness may yet be accounted for when the hormone evaluation is done.

She reported that WPA had been wonderful and paid all charges to date, for which she is truly grateful.

A post-operative check-up and the hormone tests are being carried out on 3 October. Meanwhile, Jean is thrilled at the loss of that awful soreness and thrilled at the continuing hope for a full recovery.

Follow-up – October

The vaginal progress continues and the gynaecologist had recommended one week of Sultrin vaginal cream followed by an occasional weak Betadine douche. Apparently, whilst under the anaesthetic, Jean's uterus was found to be full of residual menstrual fluids because the erosion had partially blocked the cervical opening, literally stopping menstrual blood from reaching the vagina. He cleaned it all out and did a full D&C as well as removing the erosion. Jean has now had two normal periods, heavier than in the past year and lasting a truer 5–6 days instead of dribbling for only two.

The first of the blood tests are through. Not only is she very low on iron (haemoglobin) but she also has a blood condition called esinophilia, which is an abnormality of the red blood corpuscles.

Jean is trying to overcome her natural fury that the NHS, in all their blood tests and vaginal checks, has totally failed to spot any of this. Don't forget, this current gynaecologist sends off all samples to a private laboratory for analysis. He has now twice shown her her cervix with the help of a mirror at the end of the couch. At the first consultation it was so swollen that the speculum could barely be positioned and the vagina was angrily red; but now, Jean is no longer swollen and red and can see for herself that her painfree vagina and cervix are pink and clean. She is absolutely thrilled! The tiredness continues, which at this stage is to be expected. The recent discovery of the two blood conditions will, by themselves, be making her feel dreadfully low, never mind her family of five, which must be a daily exhaustion.

Follow-up – mid-November

The hormone evaluation has come through and shows normal levels, so a major line of enquiry has been eliminated. The blood condition called esinophilia, which involves malfunction of the red corpuscles, is apparently an indicator of severe allergic reactions. Jean's mother is a proven allergy victim and Jean, under new lines of questioning relevant to allergies, reveals classic allergy reactions to dust, rabbits, chemical contact and possibly some foods. But this has not, as yet, been explored, discussed or treated within an allergy unit.

All these new enquiries have stemmed from an episode that occurred three weeks ago. Jean and Jim had gentle intercourse at 1 a.m., and at 5.20 a.m. she awoke in severe pain from the vagina. Redness was spreading out from the vagina on to the perineum, the urethra was beginning to twinge and she felt absolutely dreadful and full of fear. Since it was a Saturday, she couldn't find a VD unit open for an examination. She was reluctant to try the GP, so she instituted the water/bicarb routine and kept reasonably comfortable for some time, until she realized that the redness and swelling were not changing. By now, Sunday had arrived and, governed by fear, she commenced on some medicine-chest Amoxil antibiotic capsules of 500 mg strength. She thought she would prefer to have 250 mg rather than 500, so she opened the capsule and halved the powder, taking both amounts without the gelatinized capsule. For the first time she had no stomach upset, and during a phone call with her mother found out that she always took the capsule off for just the same reason! So Jean established an allergic reaction to the gelatin and/or the dyes.

Back to the story. On Monday, Jim suggested ringing the gynae-cologist, who was able to see her later that day since it was an emergency. In discussion of this sensitivity, Jim revealed that he had not used their normal Durex sheath for that last session of intercourse. He had run out of supplies and bought another type. Following this disclosure the gynaecologist rang up the manufac-turer, told him he had a patient who had been severely affected by the sheath manufactured by his company and asked for a complete list of the dyes, chemicals and synthetic rubber used in its manufac-turing process. The manufacturer was mightily upset and has agreed immediately to comply.

Jean's vagina changed in four hours from a normal to a highly painful and abnormal state following the use of that sheath, and it has stopped the slow recovery dead in its tracks for three weeks. Now she has a period and must wait before attempting further intercourse until it's finished.

The cervical erosion area on her cervix has responded well to the August operation but the gynaecologist is still seeing a small red patch in the middle that hasn't yet fully healed. The rest has. He thinks that some cells are deep and still active, so he is giving it two more months. If it hasn't cleared by then, he may have to cauterize it again.

The sheath business provoked another serious discussion of contraceptives. Jean and I refute the installation of a coil; the gynaecologist feels differently; Jim and I favour a vasectomy for him; Jean doesn't yet and here her strong religious feelings override, at the moment, her own welfare. She wants to be sure that God is behind such a decision, and so she and Jim are praying about it. Even with five children she still feels that it was intended for her to have six and she feels 'unfinished'; that's the only way she can explain it. Fostering and adopting are possibilities that she is at least prepared to consider. I personally feel that the vasectomy is the better bet.

Practically, I suggested douching after intercourse. The gynaecologist has already instigated douching to aid the cervical healing, but I am now suggesting its wider use after intercourse to reduce the inflammation and possible bruising, although Jim is too gentle to bruise her. I also suggested that, to stimulate better vaginal health, intercourse might happen every Saturday night around 11 p.m. so that Jean could get a full night with her feet up and resting. Intercourse at 1 a.m. on a week night and rising at 7 a.m. is not providing her with sufficient rest in her current state.

We have all been at this since May, and the latest turn of events shows more months of patience to come. None of her friends understands at all what drama, trouble and torment she is going through and just what a load of courage she has to persevere and keep on seeking. She says that I am boosting her morale no end, and for that I am pleased. I also know that this care of her would be unlikely to happen anywhere else in the world. I have talked today with an allergy specialist who in his sphere is pushing medical barriers of knowledge and asked for the best NHS allergy clinic. He gave the department of medicine at Guy's teaching hospital as being the current 'bee's knees', and Jean now has a name and the possibility of a referral letter to this allergy clinic from her now fully cooperating and marvelling GP. The gynaecologist fully approves.

I might just point out to the reader here the differences in time alone between the few patients in this book. Some have responded to ideas, self-help and treatments in two weeks; others in two months; and others, like Jean, many months. This individuality is what cystitis is all about, so can you wonder that I've never allowed group meetings! Can you wonder that some patients go for years in a state when such specialized care is required to untangle only one woman!

Follow-up – January

Step by slow step Jean's recovery is progressing. At this month's gynae examination, the remaining red patch on the cervix shows itself to have healed completely, and thankfully there is now no need for a second cauterization. The gynaecologist has made another careful examination in response to reported soreness at the very entrance of the vagina.

It is interesting to remember the state that the vagina and uterus were in on her first visit to the gynaecologist. He could hardly examine her, so heavily infected and swollen was she from the cervical erosion. As the skin has slowly recovered so Jean can now isolate, by touch, this remaining area of soreness at the entrance, which she can point to as being the spot from which soreness and pain emanate after intercourse.

Intercourse has occurred only once in the past six weeks and was of a fairly stationary nature. Jim used Durex, and although there was no trace of a general vaginal reaction as had occurred with the other sheath, Jean had her usual three-hour period next night of twingeing and soreness. She also describes it simply as 'pain at the entrance of the vagina'.

The gynaecologist, guided by Jean's fingers, then looked intently. Showing up more clearly now, surrounded by healthy pink skin, is a thin-skinned, darker patch situated by the top bone at the vaginal entrance. This patch has a history. It is called a labial graze and was a childbirth injury after Matthew was born in 1978. This piece of skin tightened so much after the birth that Jim couldn't penetrate her at all in later intercourse, so the hospital stretched it and didn't bother with anaesthetic.

The patch is, according to our gynaecologist, only 3 mm thick in flesh instead of 6–7 mm as it apparently should be. Accordingly he has prescribed Dinoestrol cream to be inserted into the whole vagina and Hormofemin cream just for the labial graze. Jean gingerly inserted some of each on the first night, expecting a reaction. There was none. She has now used them for a week and is very thrilled that the vagina has tolerated them. She feels that this, too, is also on the right track. The hormone creams will build up the vaginal health and encourage the growth of more skin cells to pad the graze.

One by one, Jean's problems are being steadily and correctly dealt with by the gynaecologist. She is feeling altogether better. Confidence is returning and with much talking to Jim and praying to God she does realize that another baby would be putting all this work at risk again. The idea of fostering becomes more appealing and can be done for many years in the future. Vasectomy is still under discussion and no longer viewed unfavourably.

The local church had a ministry of healing discussion on rejection at Christmas, and Jean came to realize that, although she had long ago forgiven her brother for the childhood sexual troubles, inside herself she was still rejecting him. The church discussions also helped her to take practical steps to heal their relationship. A long talk at Christmas has resulted in a joyousness and lifting of spirit which has lightened her mind and coincided happily with the continuous regaining of her physical health.

An even greater thrill, apparently, over Christmas was the triumphant taking of two baths! The first she has dared to take for many months because they always caused increased discharge and soreness. The big decision was how long to stay in. Jean took a mug of tea upstairs with her, washed first and then lay on in the bath until she'd drunk the tea. That was it and out she got.

She says that she has never felt so pleased with herself and those two baths were the finest Christmas present she's ever had.

Jean will continue under our gynaecologist's care until she is able to have normal reaction-free intercourse. That shouldn't be too long now. She will also keep her appointment with the allergy clinic.

Without the Western Provident Association Ltd providing funding for Jean's badly needed medical treatment, such very special care could not have been undertaken. WPA have unquestioningly paid up all the bills from day one, and now have a most grateful client who will sing their praises whenever the occasions demands. They, naturally, don't pay over and above the year's agreed contract sum, but the point is that Jean needed immediate aid and, under WPA, received it. There is no doubt that the National Health Service could not look after her. For those doubters of private medicine, including trade union officials who have their very own private hospital whilst insisting that the rest of us don't get to have it, I must ask: Was it better for Jean to remain ill within the NHS or to get well outside it?

Western Provident Association Ltd
Culverhouse
Culver Street
Bristol BS1 5JE

Tel: Bristol (0272) 273241

When Jean filled in her WPA form she had no idea of the immense amount of work of a gynaecological nature that would be implemented. WPA would not contract with her for urological work connected with cystitis but since there was then no history of gynaecological trouble they did not exclude gynaecological investigations.

My opinion of health insurance is changing with the heavily increasing charges of both Health Associations and consultants.

I would like to see both consultation and hospital fees working on a hire purchase arrangement just as home furnishings operate these days. This would be an additional form of payment to the Health Cover plans of associations like WPA – in other words, an extra choice.

CHAPTER TWELVE

Miss Alison Tippett and Ken

Alison Tippett, aged 25, was the sort of woman whom you always hope that you might be lucky enough to sit next to at an all-female lunch. Apart from looking cool and attractive in a pretty blue patterned shift dress with smart white sandals, her life is full of unusual interest and activity. Starting with hobbies, she plays squash once a week, cycles when fit each day for a short time, enjoys a swim now and again and enjoys her current boyfriend. This one, Ken, aged 30, is a full-time newspaper writer in Wales, whose hobbies include photography, cricket, football and travelling. Alison and Ken meet every other weekend or whenever possible.

In 1977 Alison went to Oxford to do a degree course at the Oxford Polytechnic in the Disasters and Settlements Unit. This unit specializes in research for aid to places in the world which have suffered any kind of natural disaster – hurricanes, famine, drought, floods, volcanic eruptions etc. It all appealed to her greatly and she returned from India in August 1983 having completed a year's fieldwork there. She lived in a small village house with a family, and at one stage in our counselling commented upon the women in that house who never wore underwear beneath their saris and always washed down with a jug of water after completing their toilet. Alison never saw precisely how they washed, but she knew they did wash.

She and Ken met at a party in October 1983, two months after her return from India, and apparently they clicked because Ken, too, had been to India.

After this exotic start, I really had to force the conversation round to the reason for her visit!

Symptoms

Cystitis – attacks of it with urethral twinges leading to pain on micturition, accelerating frequency and occasional blood loss; particularly in the last week's attack, which went up to her kidneys with temperature and malaise. Chronologically, she had one attack many years ago and then none until January 1982. Between then and April 1982, 4 months, she had 4 attacks. She broke with her current boyfriend in April 1982 and went to India for one year. From April 1982 until 1984, including the year in India, she had no boyfriends sexually and no cystitis.

From March 1984 to July 1984, once she had begun having intercourse with Ken, she had 5 attacks, one of which did not seem related to sex but rather to swimming in a public pool. Three attacks have been treated with antibiotics and two she has successfully cleared by the management procedure – water and bicarb etc.

There are no daily problems of soreness or discharge, and although she has been gynaecologically examined twice, on neither occasion was a swab taken. She has had thrush once or twice early in her university days but none since.

Urological history

Mid-stream urine specimens: Three. Two showed unknown but
    positive infections. One showed E.Coli
Antibiotics prescribed and taken.
Intravenous pyelogram: None
Cystoscopy: None

Gynaecological history

Periods began aged 15. They were slight and used up less than one packet of sanitary towels. They remain light now because of the Pill. She has not had a D&C.
One Pap (smear) test.
One check for the Pill and a diaphragm fitting.
Thrush twice between 1977 and 1979.

Contraception

Low-dose Pill. The sheath was used for a month in March 1984. In this month Alison had the first of the five current attacks of cystitis. After being on the Pill in Oxford for 18 months, she had her first four attacks, apart from the single early occurrence.

Sex

As already indicated. It's always enjoyable and, including foreplay, can last upwards of half an hour. Lubrication is good. Neither the old Oxford boyfriend nor Ken are circumcized and Alison feels that she can't check Ken's hygiene, but in the course of discussions following her visit to me, she may find an appropriate moment to mention it. She doesn't wash before sex or after.

General health

Good, although she returned from India with roundworm and giarda, which, apparently, is a digestive-system parasite. Both conditions were investigated and successfully treated at the hospital for Tropical Diseases in London.

Self-help

Alison has read both my books, uses the management of attack procedure sometimes successfully, but she does confess to not always starting it on the very first twinges. This would account for the times when infections have risen higher and needed antibiotics.

Clothing

Good. She wears dresses, skirts, no jeans, occasional tights but it's all inapplicable really, since we are dealing with proven infections.

Food intake

No notes were taken – inapplicable to infections.

Liquid intake

Intelligent. Drinks water at onset of an attack and maintains a higher intake when attack has subsided than when she is completely clear. Drinks occasional wine.

Hygiene

I took this history of hygiene immediately after the sex questions whilst Alison was with me. This was her reply and I stopped the counselling immediately:

'I do not wash after passing a stool. No, I don't wash on returning home.' And, as she had previously said, she wasn't washing before sex either. This, after reading my books and with all her MSUs showing bowel bacteria in the urine!

Upstairs in the bathroom, I took her step by step through the simple washing routine with bottle; but even on the way upstairs, the light of her error had dawned in the face of my scolding.

My suggestions – in chronological order

1 A thrush check please, in view of the recent antibiotics.
2 Ask what the results of urine tests are and specifically request the name of the bacteria and where it might have come from.
3 After swimming: shower, pass urine, drink a pint of water, and perhaps also a small amount of bicarbonate of soda to alkalize the urine and remove its normal mild acidity – a welcome mat for swimming-pool bacteria.
4 If you do start any more attacks, go to a VD/genito-urinary clinic saying that you think you may have a discharge. Reveal under questioning once in the consulting room that the urethra is twingeing. You will be vaginally examined and get the urine tested – all free.
5 Wash as demonstrated after a stool or certainly when you have returned home.
6 Wash as demonstrated after intercourse.
7 Your cystitis is being caused by perineal faecal contamination and a completely absence of washing. It should never happen again for this reason. Other reasons in your future life may arise.

My comments

A very clear-cut and extremely common case, which is why I am so pleased to include it in the book. It illustrates beautifully the fact that, whilst sex education and contraceptive education in our modern society are good, the simple hygiene so vital in achieving happy sexual health is absolutely missing. Why isn't this being taught at school and by women one to another?

Alison herself had already related sexual activity to her attacks of cystitis, but she admitted that, despite reading my books, she had still only concentrated on alleviating an existing attack. Her visit to me made her look at preventing attacks from ever starting.

The Pill might be construed by some as a precipitating factor, until you go back to the MSU results. They showed clear infection of the bladder by faecal material and attacks began 24–36 hours after intercourse. Infections require that amount of time to gain a hold following their introduction. In intercourse, faecal material can be massaged up the urethral tube, even though intercourse is taking place in the next-door vagina. What affects the vagina is also highly likely to affect the urethra. That is why I am so hot on vaginal examinations and the use of VD/genito-urinary clinics. I only wish male doctors would be able to understand this simple fact of female life more readily.

A urologist will not by nature examine the vagina and vice versa. A VD unit bears both in mind.

Alison will never again have cystitis from this cause.

Follow-up – August

Alison has seen Ken only once since our counselling. she enacted all the self-help procedures and did not start cystitis – a most encouraging sign. However, the local GP prescribed a further course of Ampicillin 'just to make sure' that the germs had gone when she went back for a clearance urine test. The test was negative but, thanks to the Ampicillin, she now has mild thrush and is going to have six days on a tube of Canesten, which she has at home. When that is finished she will go to a VD unit for a clearance check for thrush.

Alison is not seeing Ken for a weekend during this thrush episode – which is all to the good, since sexual activity could prolong the thrush and together with thrush might trigger off more cystitis.

Follow-up – late August

The following letter arrived on my desk:

I'm sorry that I haven't contacted you before now. I've a mixture of good and bad news to report.

The last time I spoke to you on the phone I suspected that I had an attack of thrush after I (sillily!!) accepted yet another course of antibiotics from my GP when these were probably unnecessary. I did use the Canesten and went along to the Westminster Hospital, Dept OP6, for a check-up. I do recommend this place – the doctors and nurses I saw were *extremely helpful* and sympathetic. The swabs proved negative as did the later cultures. So at present I am and feel, 100%!

Unfortunately, my relationship with Ken isn't so good! The odds seemed to be stacked against us from the start since he was working in Cardiff and I in London. Jobs are likely to keep us separated for much longer than we envisaged, which has put a strain on the relationship. At present, we have broken up and I think it's likely to be permanent. My recurrent cystitis certainly didn't cause this break-up but no doubt, it introduced a lot of tension which we could have done without.

As far as I know, after all your advice, I was managing to prevent my cystitis; I wish that for my own peace of mind our break up could have occurred (if at all) well after I'd banished this recurrent pest.

Thanks for your help. It has been invaluable. I feel that I now understand far more about my body and what was happening to cause my cystitis. Consequently, I can look after myself better with more control and confidence.

Yours with very best wishes and many thanks
Alison Tippett

What a shame that Alison was unable to have a few more weekends with Ken to really prove to herself that her new hygiene and bathroom routines were the answer to her cystitis. Perhaps, by the time that this book is published, she will have managed a few more guinea-pig sessions!

CHAPTER THIRTEEN
Mrs Lindy Steinbeck

Lindy Steinbeck is an American from New York and 32 years old. She has long tightly curled brown hair and is very slim, probably about size 10 and about 5 foot 6 tall. She wore a green tee-shirt and heavy cream sweater over a calf-length, full patterned skirt. Peeping from beneath this skirt were lilac-coloured leisure-wear bottoms and then socks and shoes.

She came complete with a sheaf of notes because her history of thrush is now six years old and she has conducted an exhaustive search for relief from it. Two weeks before coming to me she had married Justin, who is British, having lived with him over the past year. They had had a romantic meeting in Florence and conducted an intercontinental courtship by post, telephone and meetings.

Justin is a barrister with a professional singing interest in opera and is building a second career in London on the opera circuit.

Lindy is an expert translator from Spanish to English, and when she left New York and her parents, it was in order to go to Boston to teach Art and Spanish. She paints for a hobby at the moment and has not taught Art since moving to London. Other interests include volunteer projects for Amnesty International with her use of Spanish, and classical dancing three times a week. Justin limbers up, too, and Lindy reckons that with his lithe and compact body he'd be quite good.

So these two are in love, artistic in several ways, but having a thoroughly unsettled and miserable relationship.

Symptoms

Thrush, diagnosed – treated without success and without remission even immediately after a course of pessaries. No oral treatment has ever been prescribed. Symptoms began six years ago when she was about 27. An early spell on the Pill in her late teens did not produce thrush. An allergist has found a specific kind of candida, and although many investigations have been undertaken there is still no successful result. Symptoms are slightly relieved a few days before menstruation, but during and after they are very much worse. Irritation and curdy discharge are causing a very sore vagina and perineum. There are occasional signs of cystitis and urethral twinge-ing, especially if intercourse has been attempted.

Urological history

Urine tests are negative and taken when cystitis begins.
One cystocopy: negative.
In 1975 and 1977 she was taken into hospital in Boston to pass kidney stones comprised of calcium oxcelate. Her family has no urological or renal history.

Gynaecological history

Periods began at 13 years and were very painful for a couple of days. They were moderately heavy and lasted a good 6 days. Over the past 6 years they have lightened and now only last 3–4 days. Her hair has begun greying and she colours it regularly.
No D&Cs.
A gynaecologist in London has pronounced her well but re-commended her to a cranial osteopath for the thrush! (That's quite ludicrous and she left quickly following heavy sexually suggestive remarks. She never went to the cranial osteopath.)

Babies and pregnancies

None.

Contraceptives

Lindy was put on the Pill for a year for teenage acne. At the end of that year she also visited a naturopath who irrigated the digestive tract, and the combination of these two treatments has, Lindy says, seen off the acne completely. Since she began any kind of sex life, condoms and withdrawal have been the main forms of contraception. A diaphragm was used for 1½ years at some stage.

Sex

Absolutely miserable. There is barely any penetration, no enjoyment and it lasts minutes only. Soreness is instant and urethral involvement lasts for several days after. Genital lubrication is hampered by soreness and discharge and Lindy has found KY Jelly to sting under these circumstances, probably because the skin is so sore anyway. The couple's reaction has been to use oral sex as a second-rate substitute.

General health

No diabetes. Plenty of allergies. No operations except tonsil removal. Greying hair since spring 1982. Never needs antibiotics for anything.

Food intake

Does not eat sugar, cakes, sweets or much fruit. Does eat plenty of spicy food like curries, pepper and chilli because Justin likes these.

Liquid intake

Doesn't drink alcohol at all. Doesn't drink canned juices or Coke. Usually sticks to mineral water and had water during the counselling.

Clothing

Lindy cuts out the crotch from her leisure-wear bottoms and mostly goes without pants because she feels that she doesn't like to keep the discharge confined and pressing back around the vagina. She wears cotton tights and leotards for dancing a total of 4½ hours a week. There have been many periods of time when she has not danced during the six years of continuous thrush. She doesn't use Tampax.

Hygiene

On being taken upstairs to my bathroom for a fuller understanding on my part of how Lindy washes and a fuller understanding on her part of how I recommend washing, we found problems.

Lindy washes several times a day by sitting on the edge of the bathtub and using the handshower back to front. She holds it *behind* her and sprays upwards! Sometimes she doesn't dry herself at all, other times she uses toilet tissue to dry with. She has free-range pubic hair.

Justin rarely drinks, rarely takes antibiotics, but he does have a lot of stomach wind, which Lindy finds embarrassing but never says so. Of course, the flatulence may be due to the spicy foods.

My suggestions

1 Justin should have thrush tests.
2 Both of you should receive treatment at the same time.
3 Oral treatment, Nystatin tablets, have never been prescribed. I would recommend that you suggest this to the next doctor and ask for a four-week course of three tablets a day.
4 Dept OP6 of the Westminster Hospital functions by appointment and, like many VD units, will be careful and sympathetic on thrush.
5 We are going to 'stubble burn' for two months, 'raze the field', erase anything that could in any way be contributing to the promotion of this fungus in your body.
6 No oral, vaginal or rectal sex – no sex of any kind for two months.
7 No hand stimulation of you by Justin.
8 Cut pubic hair with scissors to ½ inch to aid air access.
9 Intercourse will cause heat and moisture.
10 Stop dancing for two months.
11 No more hot, spicy foods.
12 Stop sitting on the edge of the bath and showering back to front. Use the bottle method only.
13 I think that a check on the hormone balance is indicated here, since thrush is worse during and after a period. Also a check on the acid/alkaline levels of the vagina. Also, how heavily is the uterus invaded by thrush?
14 I gave the name of a gynaecologist who has, on a couple of past patients of mine, checked the uterus for thrush and found it necessary to pack the uterus, under anaesthetic, with gentian violet dressings. Is this another such case?
15 Periods are lighter over the last six years and thrush has worsened.
16 There is now much tension being caused by thrush. This

stress may also be affecting the hormone output and in turn leading to epithelial (skin) changes in the vagina.

My comments

After an hour or more of rummaging and casting around as broad an outlook on Lindy's thrush as possible, I turned again to the periods and the hygiene in that order.

Two things came at me together:
1 Thrush was substantially worse during and after a period.
2 Periods had lightened by a half in the six years coinciding with the onset of continuous thrush.

Additionally, Lindy then volunteered that she has had to colour her hair since spring 1982, and also that she had previously wondered about a hormonal involvement – but all doctors so far have laughed. The specialist whom I have recommended is the one who spends time in looking at all aspects of vaginal/cervical health and has also a good working knowledge of hormones. I felt that he should cover this blank area of investigations in Lindy's extensive search for help so far.

Upstairs, in the bathroom discussing hygiene, several appalling facts of Lindy's washing were discovered:
1 She doesn't use soap to remove faecal material
2 She showers too often each day
3 She showers upwards from behind
4 In doing so she propels rectal thrush forward, faecal material forward and creates a terrific bacterial/fungal mix-up
5 Thrush loves moisture – spraying is moisturizing
6 She often doesn't dry herself – more moisture
7 If she does dry the perineum, it is with toilet tissue, grains of which will be left behind to contaminate her skin.

Although Lindy has had the American edition of one of my books for three years, like so many others, she just hasn't paid attention to the washing chapter and was amazed at my demonstration up in the bathroom showing her how much harm she has been doing to herself.

Following the line on periods, my 'hunch', which can so often be right, seemed at last to be feeling more secure and centred. Of course, everything else is also important and must be attended to but unremitting thrush – no tiny breaks, even, nor response to conventional courses of treatment – is different. Lack of hormones – and she's skinny – may well be the hitherto undiscovered root cause. We'll see.

Follow-up – August

Lindy saw the gynaecologist and had an extensive check-out. Microscope analysis of the vaginal discharge showed two heavy and separate infections which have not been diagnosed by other physicians and absence of thrush. They were haemophilius and gardnerella, both very unusual and treatable with Flagyl tablets. Cryosurgery was recommended, and along with other tests was carried out in a day unit on 8 August. Lindy is now at the end of the first menstruation to occur since the operation and is waiting to see how the vagina is after that. It all takes time and we have to fit in with Nature's little timetables!

Follow-up – September

Lindy rang to report that all was marvellous after the period – no twingeing, no thrush, no stinging or irritation, but there was a whitish creamy discharge that was not giving any adverse effects. I explained that this was the non-sexually-active vagina's normal discharge. She didn't know this.

A week after the end of the period when everything was wonderful, she and Justin had some foreplay and the best four minutes of sex for well over a year. She used plenty of KY Jelly, passed urine, although not a lot, and was ecstatic! At 11 o'clock the next morning she began an attack of cystitis. She quickly rang the gynaecologist and he took vaginal swabs and urine samples – both were negative. No infections, and this could only mean, together with the short length of time between intercourse and cystitis, that the unused vagina had reacted against the now 'forgotten' act of intercourse.

Close questioning by me followed and it transpired that:
- The four minutes of intercourse had been all movement – no rests during which the unused vagina might have had
- The normal creamy discharge, which most women have and is more prevalent where intercourse is irregular, has not been gently hooked out each day. This is best done after the

bottle-washing procedure following a bowel movement. With a clean third finger, it is easily removed for the day and will prevent the mucous from travelling around the perineum as you walk. Lindy didn't know about this and will adjust her washing routine to include it.

- Her liquid intake is suspect. The gynaecologist has ordered acidity levels to be recorded on litmus paper each day.
- Lindy has announced that their postponed honeymoon is shortly to take place in Spain and will last two weeks. I have suggested the following, and I didn't like to add that I would have waited a little longer before embarking on the great adventure!

1   Liquid intake must be high
    (a) to stop dehydration in the warm weather of Spain.
    (b) to keep the uric acid in the bladder better diluted.
    (c) to have enough urine in the bladder for passing after sex.
2   Each night have a level teaspoonful of bicarbonate of soda AND a glass of water after nightly intercourse to enable a good early-morning non-acid flow of urine.
3   Have longer sessions of sex, say upwards of 15 minutes, but rest up and chat for a minute or so with Justin still inside so that the vaginal walls can relax, loosen and expand.
4   IF any twingeing starts don't wait – immediately do the management of attack. With the good washing – and she's going to use bottled water for washing in Spain – the likelihood of urinary infection is non-existent. Any twingeing is more likely to be sexual trauma because the vagina has led a sex-free existence for over a year and has probably contracted.

Lindy also needed reassuring that her original symptoms have now completely gone – no irritation, no soreness, no twingeing, no thrush, no discharge. The operation has worked; what happened after the recent sex session is something different and is temporary whilst the vagina readjusts to being used again and while she learns to aid this adjustment. We all wait with baited breath for a phone call after her honeymoon and wish her well!

Follow-up – November

Lindy's honeymoon was sex-less! The food in Spain – white bread, oil, red meat and other differences caused severe constipation. Laxatives caused diarrhoea, so her system was totally upset and she was too nervous to attempt intercourse. Had she monitored the laxatives, taking one tablet every other day, things might have been different. There was no cystitis or soreness.

Since the last follow-up she and Justin have had only one session of sex, lasting a very short four minutes. Detailed questioning revealed:

- There was no foreplay
- Oral sex was used during and after the four minutes, not before
- KY Jelly lubricant was used
- Urine was passed and she washed with cool water from the bottle
- The room was and always is without heating
- Justin sleeps naked but Lindy puts on heavy pyjamas

Lindy was sore the next morning, not during or after sex. She needed to take bicarbonate of soda and step up her liquid intake. The soreness subsided after 36 hours. She did not go to the doctor.

Vaginally speaking, there have been no infections, twingeing or soreness at all since the August operation. Thus three full months of good health are now backing our actions. Despite this tremendous improvement, Lindy is still very nervous of intercourse so she rarely allows it, and it is unnaturally short, bringing on soreness.

It will bring on soreness because of the manner in which it is undertaken. A strong talking to from me has produced her agreement to follow a regime for one month. I explained again that an unused vagina contracts and is less tolerant to the activity of intercourse when that intercourse is so rarely performed. For one month she is to:

1 Have intercourse every Saturday and Tuesday night.
2 Warm the room until she can stand naked in it without shivering.
3 Have at least 20–30 minutes of petting and relaxation before any penile penetration.
4 Reject oral sex for a while.
5 Use KY Jelly in dollops as she does at present.

6   Make sure the bowels aren't constipated. If you insert a clean finger into the vagina you can feel whether there are any faeces in the lower bowel. If you haven't passed a stool for 36 hours and you can feel hard lumps then you are probably constipated and these may encourage vaginal bruising during intercourse.

7   Abandon herself to her own excitement and orgasms and not wait for Justin to ejaculate. He will enjoy watching her pleasures.

8   Have penetration lasting for 10 minutes after the foreplay and increase on those 10 minutes over the month as vaginal toleration and elasticity improves.

9   Have fast, slow and halt spells of penile thrusts within the ten minutes of penetration, with the penis remaining inside the vagina.

10 Pass urine, poor cool water from the bottle, hook out sexual liquids from the vagina.

11 Drink a glass of water after sex to replace sweat and the expelled bladder urine so that next morning she can pass non-acidized urine.

12 Take a painkiller with this water to help calm down the excited vagina nerve-endings.

13 Maintain a good liquid intake next day. Any soreness or reaction will have started by lunchtime.

14 Return to bed from the bathroom and sleep naked next to Justin. This will heighten their body awareness and knowledge of one another, but more importantly will allow air access to cool the used vagina. Pyjamas are unsexy and air-restrictive.

Lindy readily admits that she and Justin don't 'know' one another sexually. She says that she still feels virginal and this has been heavily aided by the long experience of those nasty vaginal infections, now stopped. She is sexually inexperienced and because of the infections has now developed bad sexual habits. I have now become a sex therapist for them both, but I own quickly to having no professional knowledge in this field. If this month of simple experiment fails then I may suggest that they seek a reputable course of professional sex therapy. I have not taken such a step before. I hope that this month's regime works.

Follow-up

Lindy reports a steady improvement each time she and Justin have intercourse. The gynaecologist has also recommended that the daily vegetarian intake of onions with almost every dish be cut out. Some people are allergic to onions, and a bladder system heavily influenced by onions might be accounting for the urethral soreness in Lindy's case after sex. The vagina is well and healthy and sex is absolutely painless now. When she was first examined the vaginal infections almost prevented a full insertion of the instruments.

No onions and twice-weekly sex seem to be the final coat of icing on a very carefully baked cake! I regard Lindy as well; so does she.

CHAPTER FOURTEEN

Lady Calista

It was early morning when the car came off the motorway. The driver knew nothing about it; he was already asleep, lulled by the warmth, the purr of the engine, the empty roadway and the drinks at the party in London. His young wife of four years didn't know too much about it either, but she alone woke up. He never did.

A widow at 26 with three tiny children, Lady Calista's first hazy memories of those events began in Stoke Mandeville Hospital for Spinal Injuries. She feels that the coping with new widowhood was eased into second place by an immediate new life which the accident had now imposed upon her; a life commanded totally by the broken body and severed spinal cord which have glued her to a wheelchair for the rest of her days. So far, she has battled for 20 years and is even now only 46.

There are braver people, she says, with even worse disabilities, in their wheelchairs. She's right, but that doesn't detract from the enormous welling-up of sympathy and shuddering horror, which is what we able-bodied people considerately feel for such victims. To spend three hours with such a person within their own home, not the protective custody of a hospital environment, is to catch a flash only of just what it means to sit when others walk, to sit when others stand, to sit when others rush around.

Married at 22, widowed and paralysed at 26, her God is the Roman Catholic God who blessed and comforted her before the accident with 3 children, as if apologizing in advance. The family was moneyed, and cushioned with its cash the particular terror bereaved and disabled people have of being poor. A two-storeyed house was found and gadgeted. Everything on the ground floor is at her level; gates work by electric buttons, the car is carefully adapted, and upstairs is a marvellous young husband-and-wife team, which cleans, odd-jobs and gardens. They and their two young babies add absolute normality and cheerfulness to the sparkling, colourful rooms, which the dog patrols with territorial confidence. Much thought has gone into providing the right home and an uplifting spirit.

Her spirit *has* to be redoubtable; depressions *must* be short; because there are years and years to go yet. It takes Lady Calista two hours to dress every morning. She must clean up after lying in puddles of her own uncontrolled urine, leaking despite the padding; wet night-wear has to be removed and laundered; bowels emptied manually with plastic-gloved fingers; the muck has to be cleaned up afterwards – one's own dignity preserved; and then the tiring task of dressing and breakfasting, all before turning her mind away from caring for the wasted body to deal with other tasks, duties and pleasures.

The body is a discussed subject – much discussed, apparently, between the paralysed – in the kind of detail that none of us could believe or imagine. Nothing embarrasses them, nothing is too private to share with another. They have their jargon, they know names of bones and mucles, of side-effects and operations, of equipment and gadgets that never enter our lives. Yet with all of this, and the underlying tragedy of each and every wheelchair victim, should come the sure knowledge that their example of doggedness is inspirational and comforting to those others of us who feel cast down at times under far less trying conditions.

Lady Calista is a complete paraplegic and an incomplete tetra-plegic – that is to say, she is paralysed from the third thoracic vertebra down, which was the point at which her spinal cord was severed, roughly breast-high. Her arms, head and shoulders move, but one hand, now withered, indicates that possibly her neck also was partly broken. She can eat and drink quite normally without holding aids and 'by magic', as she says, her stomach digests food and drink with the internal organs seemingly managing pretty efficiently. Bowels and bladder have no action of their own.

There is no feeling from the chest down, but when Lady Calista tells her GP that she can 'feel' aching in her thighs and the small of her back during an attack of cystitis, he dismisses it. It is, after all, a technical impossibility! Eight years ago the jerking and spasmodic movements which her deadened body made became increasingly and embarrasingly severe. Activities outside the home were curtailed and her surgeon decided to do an alcohol block. The spinal cord was surrounded with alcohol to isolate jerks and keep the body still. This worked well, but just recently minor jerking has started again.

Frequent visits for body maintenance and appraisal are made to Stoke Mandeville. The marvellous surgeon who dealt with her for many years has gone to a unit in Oswestry, so Lady Calista sees various doctors now who, of course, all have great knowledge but maybe haven't the bonding which inevitably occurs between doctor and patient in the early life-saving days after any accident of such magnitude.

Two years ago when she was in Stoke Mandeville for some further maintenance work, the bladder was defying the normal stimuli of stroking and tickling at the base of the pubis to encourage it to empty. The attendant nursing staff resorted to over-heavy hand pressure in an attempt to squeeze and force the urine out. Lady Calista says that she can date the start of real urinary infections to that time. A subsequent bladder scan showed a bulge, possibly a diverticulum, on the top edge of the bladder, which had never been noticed before in 18 years of regular tests. Nor in those 18 years had she ever had a urinary infection – unusual in a paralysed person and lovely for her. But now urinary infections are regular and occurring every 8 to 9 weeks.

I visited her at home to throw any relevant help or light upon the problem. I also went to learn from her.

Symptoms

Attacks of cystitis noticeable only to her as cloudy, smelly urine and frequency. Although there is no pain for her, she can occasionally 'feel' an ache in the small of her back and down her thighs. Bacteria found in urine tests are E.Coli, psuedomonas or a proteus. Kidney function is good generally. There is no vaginal discharge, but constant attention has to be paid to a labia pressure sore to keep it under control. Urinary infections began in earnest two years ago. She has no thrush.

Urological tests and history

She has had most careful monitoring and much urological work done at Stoke Mandeville. Some of this work includes:

MSUs: Lots, and have shown bacteria for the last two years. Antibiotics are prescribed.

IVPs: Every other year for 18 years, but now every year since recurrent infections set in.

Dilatations: Two in the 1970s.

Micturating cystogram: Summer 1983. Normal.

An undated cystoscopy and bladder washout.

Bladder scan to show the volume of urine that the bladder can hold. This scan, done in 1984, was the first test which showed the bulge/diverticulum and it was done the day before a holiday, following which no further investigation took place on this newly discovered condition.

For 18 months Lady Calista has taken phenoxybenzamine tablets, which aid the sphincter valve to relax and allow easier manual expulsion of urine. These caused depression and she wished she'd asked to come off them earlier. Whilst under their influence, and after some pressure from her daughter, she agreed to see a psychiatrist. After consultations he came to the conclusion that she was mentally normal and healthy but suggested that the tablets were the root of the depression. She came off them, proved him right and felt that all the talking was a marvellous release and help anyway.

Gynaecological history

Periods began aged 14 years and were painful but not very heavy. They eased in the late teens.

1981   A D&C for heavy clotting.

Periods are a real burden when you sit in a wheelchair. With the incontinent bladder and the monthly bleeding she feels a real mess and can't wait for the menopause. No other gynae work has been done.

Babies

One girl, 1960, 7lbs. Easy birth but had forceps, episiotomy and stitches.

One boy, 1962, 9lbs. The episiotomy ripped and required more stitching.

One girl, 1963, 8lbs. The best delivery. Episiotomy held and stitching was minimal.

Sex

The four years of her marriage were lovely. That is all the meaningful sex life that Lady Calista has ever had. There was a tetraplegic at Stoke Mandeville with whom she shared an attraction, but he was married and she refused to contemplate any liaison.

General health

Paralysis apart, a strong constitution lies within the body and illness is rare. She stopped smoking last year and her weight is about right, but abdominal muscles have no tone at all and she now has the common 'paraplegic paunch'.

Liquid intake

She drinks about three pints of water a day on Stoke Mandeville's instructions. Four or five times a week wine or other alcohol is drunk.

Diet

Is good English and contains nothing weird.

Washing

One of my main interests in the visit was to see her explaining her hygiene. Bowels are emptied by hand a couple of times a day. Other para/tetraplegics evacuate on average every two days.

Lady Calista has an ordinary bathroom with none of the expensive equipment that the other wheelchair victim in this book has. A wheelchair friend advised her to reposition the handbasin by the lavatory and she did so. Getting in the bath takes too long, she says, and the shower unit fixed on the wall has never been used because it's all too much effort. Instead she remains in the wheelchair and strip-washes each morning at the basin.

Every bowel evacuation requires considerable clearing away and washing afterwards.

Donning plastic gloves, she reaches into the rectum and pulls out any gathered faecal material. Most drops into the loo but much of the softer stuff remains on the gloves and must be contaminating the taps and the basin, she thinks. There are two soft sponges with which she then soaps and cleans the entire perineum. Being without a sense of feeling she cannot judge whether the sponges are touching the vaginal and urethral orifices, but presumes they are because she doesn't clean systematically. The sponges are rinsed and used for removing the soap. She gets so sick and tired of it all that she isn't absolutely scrupulous each time. After towel-drying the perineum, incontinence pads are fixed inside clothing.

The lavatory seat has a brown rubber air-cushion on top to protect her delicate skin from pressure and this, too, must bear faecal contamination. Everything looks clean and she obviously makes a considerable effort to keep the bathroom sweet-smelling and pleasant.

All these routines have been practised for 20 years, only the last two of which have seen real urinary tract infections.

My suggestions

1 What about checking up on the bulge/diverticulum to see if it is retaining stale urine and encouraging flare-ups of bacterial infection?

2 Don't agree to dilatations without careful discussion and your own full understanding. Dilatations cause scarring and scarred tissue loses tone.

3 Discuss with Stoke Mandeville the possibility of alkalizing the urine each night with one level teaspoonful of bicarbonate of soda to reduce the acid 'food' level for sustaining bacterial growth.

4 Try antisepticizing the basin and taps AFTER the initial bowel evacuation but BEFORE you start on the actual washing.

5 Rinse the antiseptic off with a jug of hot water so that it can't in any way be transferred to your skin and set up a reaction.

6 Ponder upon removing the handbasin taps and substituting

a small corner unit arrangement of taps and handshower so that this could reach to the lavatory and be used for perineal washing.

7. (a) Soap the back passage only, either with hands or with a soapy flannel. The sponges can't be boiled and will always hold microscopic E.Coli.

   (b) Wash hands.

   (c) With a flow of water either from a plastic bottle or jug or newly installed hand shower, rinse off the entire perineum from front to back whilst remaining on the lavatory.

   (d) If for any reason point (c) is impossible, e.g. being in a strange bathroom, take a good supply of flannels and use in strict order:

     1 urethral/vaginal orifices
     2 anal orifice

   (e) Dry the perineum in strict order:

     1 vagina
     2 anus

   with a small towel or another flannel. A big towel is unwieldy and unnecessary.

8. Cut pubic hair to ½ inch. This will improve hygiene and air access to the perineum, especially for the pressure sore.

9. Simply drop any used flannels into a special saucepan and boil them whilst you're doing any kitchen work.

10. Have a month or two on Surgeon Captain Cleave's natural yoghurt plan to reduce intestinal E.Coli and see what happens.

My comments

I had to confine my thoughts several times just to dealing with suggestions for urinary help. There was so much else to discuss for a fuller understanding of Lady Calista's life-style, but time prohibited.

In talking flannels and not the famed bottle-washing method I had to take two of her physical restrictions into account:

1 She always needs one hand to steady her flopping body on the loo. So it would be difficult to hold a bottle of water *and*

fiddle around the cracks and crevices with the other, which in any case is withered.

2 Her legs and thighs also need to be held apart.

A light showerhead could possibly be an answer. She could lean back on the low lavatory cistern, use her good hand to hold her thighs apart and let the withered hand hold the light showerhead. This would considerably improve upon the messy business of the contaminated sponges currently used.

Her comment about using this process for 18 years without trouble was very valid, but she also could have ageing skin, just like the rest of us, which doesn't fight off bacteria so well. That, I suggested, was one possible reason, but the main one, I feel, is the possibility of that bulge/diverticulum harbouring stale bacteria in the trapped urine. Now, removing as much external contamination as possible would certainly help; but Stoke Mandeville may provide a more permanent and easy result with surgical work on the bulge. She took both points.

Lady Calista well recognizes that her basin and taps must be faecally contaminated and only she knows how much.

The local supermarket is now stocking a natural ewe's milk yoghurt from Greece and a good half pint of that a day for a month or so might help reduce gut E.Coli levels.

She gave me three hours of her time, which I much appreciated. It's quite possible that, being so sick of all the daily work which she undertakes on the paralysed body, she will lack sufficient determination to revise her hygiene, and this would be very understandable. But what I am suggesting is only a revision not an addition, and is definitely worth a bit of concentration.

It will be interesting to see if Stoke Mandeville come up with their side of manipulating an improvement in the urinary infections.

Follow-up – February

Since my visit, no appointment has been kept at Stoke Mandeville Hospital. Lady Calista likes to keep away until a visit is essential. She has, though – much to my delight since I didn't feel that she could be bothered for various reasons – revised her perineal washing. She has taken to propping one leg onto the wheelchair as she sits on the lavatory, so that this action holds her thighs apart. She leans her trunk back against the cistern and then has her good arm and hand free to wash with. Evacuation of faeces from the bowel is now done with 4–5 changes of plastic glove on her right hand. None of these gloves touches the basin and taps but is discarded when messy. The taps have been carefully disinfected and the basin also. The massive faecal contamination of basin and taps has ended.

One sponge still soaps the anus but she restricts it to that opening only. She rinses the sponge off under the tap and then wipes the anus carefully several times with the rinsed sponge. Then she soaps by hand, not sponge, the front part in case any faecal material has strayed forwards.

Next she fills a small holdable plastic bottle with tap water and pours several warm bottlefuls down over the front part. Some of this will also be running off beyond the anus but she can't feel it. Anyway, it doesn't really matter since the bottled water is cleaning the urethral and vaginal orifices very well, and that is the area where we wish to prohibit the invasion of bowel bacteria.

Since our meeting 8 weeks ago she has, after a week of antibiotics for the then present urinary infection, been quite clear of smelly or infected urine. She has had two periods in that time and each passed safely without a problem of infection. This is the longest time without a urinary infection that she has gone in the last two years since the bulge was first noted. You can tell that she's pleased and she's saving up the good news to tell Stoke Mandeville at a later, opportune time.

She feels that perhaps, as with the able-bodied female patient, male doctors can't be bothered with very simple information – and at the right moment she might just hint at that to them!

She also thinks that it might be a good idea if I visit some mixed para/tetraplegics in their homes and revise their hygiene, and form a helpful booklet for this long suffering group of men and women. Maybe next year!

Follow-up

Ten months have now passed and no urinary or kidney infections have occurred. Lady Calista puts the success down entirely to my visit, the plastic bottle of flowing water and the glove changes.

CHAPTER FIFTEEN

Mrs Renee Bigsby

Renee Bigsby is 45 years old, petite, with short, stylishly cut fair hair and an attractively made-up face. Her own hand-crotcheted white top looked stunning with her complexion and contrasted well over the sleek black corduroy trousers. She hadn't travelled far, only from south London, and she'd brought a girlfriend with her.

The girlfriend was equally vivacious and after a moment's discussion it became clear that both women were very good friends and sitting in on the counselling was not going to cause any difficulties. They knew one another well because they both worked in the same beauty salon, Renee being the receptionist/shampooist and her friend a stylist. Women's beauty parlours spawn intimacies and confidences, so I dare say that the friend knew all about Renee's problems.

Divorce had come Renee's way three years ago, but Bob had also arrived to fill the gap even though he doesn't live in. Bob works for the gas board and has rough, calloused hands which, both women chuckled, were enormous and always cold! Apparently his circulation is not too good, poor man, and the hands are permanently white and freezing!

Renee isn't sporty; she only walks to work – literally across the street! She may read or knit sometimes but has no other interests apart from the salon, Bob, eating or drinking out and shopping. She has two grown-up daughters, one married and 24 years old, the younger 18 and still living at home.

Symptoms

Burning skin and a heavy dragging feeling when she passes urine – so severe that she has to hold on to something for a few seconds to catch her breath. It is some time before she can straighten herself. The burning has been called cystitis, but she doesn't actually have attacks. These painful symptoms occur every time she passes urine, and she had purposely not drunk a lot so that she wouldn't have to go to the lavatory on her visit.

She has no thrush and has been well and frequently examined. Her skin, she thinks, is not tender; she has no hot flushes; no pains in the joints; no problems sleeping; but she is extremely fatigued and tired, possibly from being in pain yet still doing a 9–5 standing job in the salon. These symptoms – burning, dragging and fatigue began after a hysterectomy and are definitely worsening. She never had any bladder problems before.

Urological history

All urine tests are negative – no bacteria ever found – but antibiotics were given two years ago, promptly causing thrush, which she so hated that she has refused to take any more, quite rightly.

She has not seen a urologist, nor has she had a kidney X-ray.

Gynaecological history

Periods began at 14 years and have been trouble-free. Contraception has mostly been the coil in recent years and it suited her very well, but a second one was not so successful. The first coil was inserted during an operation called a cone biopsy, which was done in response to discovering cancer of the uterus. The treatment and the coil were very successful through to March 1982. In that March the old coil was removed routinely, but on the smear taken at the time, more cancer was discovered, and it was decided to do a hysterectomy. The night before the operation, in April 1982, the coil was removed. After the hysterectomy, Renee haemorrhaged, and a second catheter was inserted. This catheter caused almost instant discomfort and Renee dates her symptoms from that time.

Sex

Sporadic and not necessarily happening each week. She enjoys intercourse and finds it quite comfortable during the half-hour or so of its duration.

General health

Quite good otherwise, except for the tiredness and fear of future cancer, but she leads a regulated and cheerful life and couldn't imagine herself behaving any differently.

Diet

Amazingly, Renee's usual alcohol intake remains unmoved by her urinary discomfort and at weekends she drinks scotch and lemonade to the tune of four a night. Wine is drunk with weekend meals, and maybe lager, too. She doesn't drink during the week.

She mostly eats fresh meat and vegetables but finds that tomatoes, strawberries and soft fruit increase the burning quite considerably.

Clothing

Not very good really, e.g. the trousers; but Renee's trouble dates from a certain time and a definite event, so I have to assume that trousers have absolutely nothing to do with it and disregard the clothing.

My suggestions

1 Ask her friendly lady GP for another referral letter to the London teaching hospital which has done all the previous work. Her surgeon has now left, but I feel that she should remain in the same place and have tests on hormone levels.
2 If for any reason she does not return to that hospital, I gave her the name of another London teaching hospital which has a menopausal clinic so that the GP could refer her there.
3 The trouble *only* began after the hysterectomy, and it's getting worse. All other factors like clothing, diet, hygiene (no infections have ever been found) become insignificant. Leaving off the scotch wouldn't change anything in her case.

My comments

They're very short and simple. I can't help this patient directly. All her life, her routines were having no adverse effects upon her body, nor did she suddenly change them overnight in April 1982.

Her GP feels that some damage occurred during the catheterization, and this is a possibility. But she is also complaining of great fatigue and I would rather plump for sorting out the hormones before submitting to the rigours of urological investigation. The GP is sympathetic and helpful; Renee has full confidence that cooperation will continue, and presumably the GP will get around to investigating any possible urological damage sometime!

Having stated that I can't help this patient and explained my reasons for saying so, I must, of course, point out that no one in the teaching hospital or the medical centre has mentioned hormones, so I have instigated a new line of investigation which will hopefully yield further light on the trouble.

Follow-up – November

Renee rang, following a morning appointment at the menopause clinic whose name I gave. Her GP wrote a referral letter straight away and there was a six week wait. After asking questions set on a pre-printed form, the Sikh doctor asked extra questions about the catheterization which was done after the hysterectomy. Renee, until that moment, hadn't mentioned her feelings about a connection with the catheter. She told him of the haemorrhage and the second catheter insertion, explaining that it had hurt badly and that the surgeon had found difficulty in placing it properly. The Sikh doctor then implied that it was not unknown for the bladder neck to be damaged during catheter insertion and he wanted her to see another doctor, still within his clinic, who deals in such matters.

The Sikh doctor didn't examine her but he took two blood samples. Renee didn't ask their purpose. She now waits for these results and a second appointment. Meanwhile, following a bout of severe pain which felt like wind and for which she had to take two days off work, Renee reports a whole week of feeling perfectly well – no bladder pain at all, which is the first time since the hysterectomy. This is quite inexplicable and we will wait to see how long the remission lasts.

Follow-up – mid-February

The bad pain has returned and her remission ended. Renee kept her appointment at the London teaching hospital to see a genito-urinary specialist. This is the first time that she has been examined urologically. She was asked first thing to drink 500 mls of water and walk, especially up and down stairs, to encourage that liquid to go through to the bladder. This was in preparation for the first part of a full urodynamic investigation to be carried out without anaesthetic. Had she been given any anaesthetic, local or general, she would not have been able to respond to commands with normal muscular movements.

A urodynamic investigation measures, amongst other things, bladder muscle reaction, any urinary retention, any uncontrolled sphincter valve action, the urinary flow, and how much urine the bladder can hold comfortably. Of the 500 mls of water drunk, Renee only passed 420 mls.

On the couch in the investigation room, Renee was wired up to a television set and results were fed off into panels of instruments. A tube was passed into her rectum and linked up to a bag of water on a stand. Another tube was inserted into the urethra and up into the bladder so that the bladder could be filled with a special water solution. Renee was told to say when she couldn't bear any more of this solution. In awful discomfort and holding off from screaming, she spoke out at 320 mls and the specialist said, 'Are you really sure?' He still had most of the second bag of water solution left to empty into the tube. The next command was to 'let go and flow', which Renee did – but then she was asked to stop and this she only managed with slowness and great difficulty.

It also took time, on command, to start the flow from her bladder again. This test showed a very sluggish waterflow, and Renee says that she's often embarrassed in public lavatories when a queue builds up outside because she takes so long to get going and to complete the bladder-emptying.

The amount of pain that Renee was in during the tests, according to the specialist, was abnormal, especially on the efforts to insert the tube into the bladder opening. He says that he has seen other patients with catheter damage to the bladder neck when loose tissue had to be removed, because it was obstructing the clean flow of urine from the bladder into the urethral tube and affecting the amount of urine able to be held. Although Renee has no history of infection, such an obstruction would be likely to harbour bacteria and encourage infection.

The specialist could see on the television screen a definite obstruction to the bladder neck and feels that this is quite possibly torn or damaged skin tissue stemming from the catheterization directly after Renee's hysterectomy.

Renee was in great pain after the investigations and felt very faint and groggy. After a rest she was driven home, where she had to deal with the urethral and bladder reaction to the instrumentation. Passing urine was agonizing, and even with a heavily increased liquid intake, potassium citrate and Panadol, two days elapsed before the pain started to subside and the shock to the bladder and urethra decrease.

A letter has gone off to another specialist with the urodynamic results, and Renee has to wait for a date of admission to hospital for surgery to remove the obstruction – under a general anaesthetic, she's thankful to announce!

Renee is instinctively 'content' with all of this. She herself knows that the trouble began immediately after the hysterectomy and is convinced that the pain began with that catheterization. We must hope and pray that a 'new boy' is not given the task of operating. After all this trouble she deserves a master surgeon not an apprentice.

As for the state of her hormones, no further work has been done and the GP has not revealed any results from the menopause clinic notes. The great tiredness and fatigue has gone because the hairdressing salon has closed down and therefore Renee is at home, unemployed but rested.

The menopause clinic which I suggested she attend has been extremely thorough; they completed a fuller view of Renee's case from the urological point of interest, which had not been undertaken before, and found a reason for her constant pain which fits in with Renee's feelings about it, too.

For myself, acting as it were as an impartial investigator, I have much satisfaction just from my simple but specific referral, which has jogged the professionals into such fruitful activity, and I applaud their broadmindedness, especially that of the friendly GP who recommended Renee to me.

Well done everyone, and good luck to Renee in obtaining a swift and successful operation!

CHAPTER SIXTEEN

Mrs Gillian Varney

Mrs Varney had only received my books two days before visiting me and had already made a note of the hygiene procedures which were quite different to hers. She had come a long way to see me, from way up in Lincolnshire, on the bleak east coast. It's a lengthy and arduous journey if you're not well, but some neighbours visiting London to return their daughter to college had suggested a lift.

Gillian arrived in one piece and her friends, although offered hospitality in my house, declined and remained outside in their car. A tall, well-built woman of 34, Gillian smiled easily. Her clear complexion, still shaded by summer sun, was complemented by red cheeks and naturally curly brown hair. She wore a beige heavy cotton skirt and toning light wool blouse, with beige sandals and bare legs.

She was a little restless in my armchair, but was relaxed and eager for the discussion. She had previously sent to me by post a six-page round up of her problems, but I hadn't looked at it. Each patient sees her problem from within the wood and counts each tree, but I walk around the wood mostly disregarding the bushes and trees, trying to see the main paths and strands. Perhaps the analogy of a maze is better – I don't walk through the patient's maze I look at it, as it were, from a helicopter, and reading Gillian's history would have masked my overall view. But I do always like to know any bacterial findings either from the urine or from vaginal mucous.

Gillian married John in 1966 when she was only 17, and they had two children – the first in 1968 and the second in 1970. By 1976, after 9 years of marriage, they were divorced. For 5 years she was a one-parent family and, except for a six-month period at the end of those 5 years, she had had no sexual relationships with anyone.

At the start of that six-month period she had a coil fitted and started cystitis. This relationship ended and, by wonderful chance, she met James a few weeks later in March 1981 and he has become her common-law husband. They have now been together for 3½ years.

James is mad on sport, and so was Gillian until poor health forced her to stop. Sports include cycling, squash, badminton and skating, and they are enjoyed regularly. James plays squash and badminton several times a week and Gillian used to join him, but is not well enough now.

Having married at such an early age, Gillian had no career training and never worked at all before the wedding. Upon her divorce she entered the temporary worlds of house-cleaning, tailoring, bar work and decorating, *and* she cycled to and from the jobs. At times she had two jobs – one in the day, one at night – ran her own little home and the two children, and cycled everywhere! Here was an energetic, life-loving woman being held back now by a health problem.

Symptoms

Frequent vaginal and bladder infections with symptoms of burning, low pelvic pain, high backache; no headaches, no vomiting. Passing urine early in the morning hurts and it can now also feel worse near a period.

Thrush occasionally after antibiotics.

It all began from the time that a coil – the Lippes Loop – was fitted in March 1980. *Never* before that time had Gillian ever had cystitis or vaginal trouble, except a touch of bruising on her honeymoon in 1966. Immediately after the fitting of the coil, symptoms began and were aggravated by intercourse with the boyfriend of six months and, later, with James. James has often had bladder infections since beginning his relationship with Gillian. Her swabs and urine cultures always showed E.Coli, but since her 1983 hysterectomy some cultures are coming back negative. Four days before seeing me more cultures for an arousal of symptoms showed extensive E.Coli in the urine and the vagina.

Urological history

MSUs: Unnumbered since 1980 and always show E.Coli; some had extra streptococci. Since 1983 some cultures have been negative.

IVP: Completely clear in 1982 except for signs of inflammation which one would expect.

Cystoscopy: In March 1982, and again showed signs of regular inflammation. The hospital wanted to do bladder wash-outs but appointments got mixed up and the wash-outs never materialized.

Antibiotics: Thousands.

Gynaecological history

Periods began at 14 years and have always been excellent. E.Coli has been found on all vaginal swabs since 1980.
E.Coli-infected Fallopian tubes were removed in 1982 by a private surgeon.
The uterus became heavily infected with E.Coli and was removed in June 1983; so was the left ovary, also riddled with the same germ and having caused much trouble.
No D&C.

Contraception

During the 9-year marriage Gillian used the Pill and the sheath. She had no vaginal or urethral trouble.
In March 1980 a Lippes Loop – intra-uterine device/coil – was inserted by the Family Planning Association and there were no technical problems or pain. This coil – her one and only – was removed in March 1982. After the 1983 hysterectomy there was naturally no need for further contraception but the doctor has advised James to use a sheath in view of the extensive E.Coli infections.

Sex

Not much! Gillian and James have had two sessions in the last four weeks and would dearly love to return to their early sex life of several times a week.

Babies (from her marriage)

One girl, born 1968. Excellent labour half an hour.
One boy, born 1970. Born at home so fast that there was no time to get to the hospital. No stitches at all.

James

He has had several courses of antibiotics and has also had to have a cystoscopy for bladder infections. Gillian couldn't help but point to the source of his infections being herself.

General health

This would be good without the last three years, and certainly she looks very robust. She had her appendix removed during the hysterectomy, and when she was 21 had her varicose veins stripped for cosmetic purposes.

Life-style

She started married life in a caravan, then moved into a tiny cottage, and then into the modern three-bedroomed terrace house where she still lives. She does not have a bidet and only minor alterations like a storm-porch have been added to the house.

Liquid intake

This used to be quite average, but since 1983, after the hysterectomy and the constant fear of kidney damage, she has drunk 10 pints of liquid a day. She does pass an equivalent amount, too; I checked. Her doctors have made her cut down the 10 pints to 7–8 and would like it reduced further. It's one thing to drink a lot during an actual attack and confine it to the three hours or so, but it's quite another to activate the kidneys excessively over a long timespan. No alcohol is ever drunk.

Diet

Gillian doesn't eat curries, chilli or spicy foods. She does eat fruit, but not in quantity, maybe an apple or orange a day. In any case, the diet is irrelevant because the problem is active infection. The GPs do say, though, that she has a very acid system.

Hygiene

Up in the bathroom she described her own routines:
- baths each evening
- passes a stool each morning

- does not use any soap on the perineum at all
- washes the perineum with a wet flannel, which is changed each day

My suggestions (exactly as I wrote them down during counselling and requested Gillian to show to her GP.)

1 Hygiene is suspect. E.Coli from the morning bowel action is present through to and possibly even beyond bath time at night.

2 Night time acidity?

3 Acidity?

4 Always use soap on the rectal orifice after passing a stool and remember my bathroom demonstration.

5 Remember to wash exactly as I showed you.

6 With such severely infection-impregnated skin, the self-help may take longer than usual to show benefits.

7 The burning that is happening now since the June 83 hysterectomy might be being caused by lowering hormone levels.

8 Suggest hormone evaluation. If necessary, treatment may be by Dinoestrol cream and/or tablets.

9 Find out whether a menopause clinic exists in Lincolnshire to which you could request a referral.

10 Finish this latest course of antibiotics and keep a careful watch out for thrush. Have clearance urine and vaginal checks.

11 No doubt at all that the coil started it all and it should have been discussed following the first-ever discovery of E.Coli in the vagina.

12 Two things are now encouraging E.Coli to remain troublesome:
   (a) Daily 'topping up' of E.Coli by poor hygiene
   (b) Lowering hormone levels and reduced skin quality following ovary and uterus removal.

13 Always have swabs done whenever you are suspicious.

14 Books on hysterectomy/menopause would help explain a lot to you.

15 Dr Bilton! Could you please help on the hormone check?

My comments

What an appalling state of affairs! That no one removed that coil with its string harbouring E.Coli, nor even mentioned in those two years that the coil does often harbour infections, is a travesty of medical awareness. That Gillian has actually had to have such major surgery and has now even lost the chance to have James's children at age 34 – just because of E.Coli infections WHICH ARE STILL HAPPENING, is beyond words. It is a tragedy; it is medical mismanagement of an extremely serious nature, and one London gynaecologist full of disbelief ended by saying that if this really was true, and there is no reason at all to suppose that it is not, then litigation would appear to be indicated and certainly would be if this had happened in America.

Her doctors, except Dr Bilton, who told her to phone me and suggested that she might benefit from self-help (pity he didn't suggest it much earlier!) damn well knew where E.Coli comes from – the bowels – and have not taken minutes to discuss hygiene nor remove that disastrous coil. The string of the coil, which Gillian rightly could feel, provided a harbour for bacterial invasion from her bowels, which, without the coil string, had remained trouble-free until 1980.

In the past years of my counselling, there have been a handful of patients – such as the lady who suffered severe damage to her bladder during a routine sterilization and could hardly stand for the pain, which never stopped – who should have sought legal advice. I add Gillian to that handful.

My thoughts on the acidity – some people do have excessive acidity, not necessarily caused by dietary excesses, but in such cases a bowl of stewed plums or of fresh soft fruit could tip the bladder urine into a 'burning' situation. Obviously antibiotics are not the answer – just some bicarbonate of soda (unless there is any heart or blood-pressure trouble) and extra water will reduce the acidity level.

E.Coli will not survive in an alkaline OR a highly acidic urine. It likes a nice moderately acid environment. The vagina and normal bladder/urethra mucous are just right. In addition, Gillian's constantly inflamed and infected skin provides an extra encouragement for this nasty bacteria, which has, since the coil, invaded and permanently inhabited her entire pelvic region. Whereas you can regulate the bladder urine's pH (acidity or alkalinity measure) it is not possible to regulate the pH of the vagina, ovaries, Fallopian tubes and uterus by drinking copious amounts of water. Antibiotics and hygiene are the only answer during an actual attack.

E.Coli multiplies by itself every 12.5 minutes, so you can imagine how much it must have been enjoying itself on the string of her coil, unrestrained by any hygiene measures and continuing upwards, ever upwards. She herself topped up the levels each day with fresh E.Coli from the bowels and spread it around on her wet flannel. Intercourse helped, too, with the massaging movements and failure to wash properly after sex. James soon started to harbour it from the coil string and her infected skin. The doctor was wise to advise him to use the sheath.

The danger to him and his kidneys lies within the large prostate gland at the base of the penis, which is so intricate that any sort of infection is difficult to fully dismiss.

I took Gillian in minute detail plus reasons through the bottle-washing hygiene procedure, distinguishing for her the difference between that used after passing a stool and that used after intercourse. She felt the change in water temperature as I regulated it first for after a stool and secondly, cooler, for after intercourse. She has never inserted her finger into the vagina to cleanse it out after intercourse and I strongly suggested that she should do so. Nor has she ever used soap on any part of the perineum. I explained why it MUST be used after passing a stool on the rectal orifice to remove the greasy faecal material left in microscopic amounts after using toilet paper. Soap must NOT be used on the urethral and vaginal orifices.

Gillian is desperately worried about her kidneys. I feel that the liquid intake is protecting them by flushing them constantly and making it more difficult for E.Coli, in its rising process, to actually invade the tissue structure and settle. No doubt it's trying to, because she shivers when major flare-ups occur. Now that she has seen me and is commencing excellent hygiene, the kidneys are in less danger. It is interesting to note that she couldn't stop it rising up the reproductive organs, and it is they that have been so irrevocably damaged that they have had to be removed. You can't flush out the entire reproductive system! The latest antibiotics and the new hygiene both coinciding is very fortuitous. When the antibiotics, which hopefully are strong enough and lengthy enough, have worked, she will have stopped 'topping up' her daily E.Coli levels, so we will wait with bated breath to see what happens.

At least she knew the name of the bacteria and regularly had swabs and MSUs. I do wonder why so many women won't stand their ground and *insist* on knowing the name of their own germs!

There are all sorts of bacteria which can give very nasty urinary symptoms and whose original sources of habitation provide clues as to how they have arrived in your body. You must always ask the name and always ask where they come from.

Gillian's hysterectomy has not 'done away' with her problems – rather, the operation has added to them! The loss of the one ovary and the uterus will very likely have lowered the hormone levels, and this can cause its own brand of twingeing and burning, and account for the negative urine results of late. So I do hope that Dr Bilton pulls on his own local strings and tries to make up a little bit for the great suffering that his profession has largely imposed upon this energetic young woman.

In July 1984, the other GP whom Gillian visits suggested a course of psychiatric treatment for her! She refused. Now how can that man line up constantly proven E.Coli infections with 'something in the mind'?

If anyone requires a course of anything in this affair it's that GP, who needs a revisionary course in gynaecology and bacteriology! Beyond that, I'm largely speechless now, and we'll see what transpires from the follow-up. I do wish, though, that Gillian could afford to put herself in the hands of more competent doctors.

Follow-up – mid-November

This is disappointing. Gillian has had no further MSUs or vaginal swabs taken in the month since she saw me, but even so, two further courses of antibiotics – five days each – have been taken. She's all right when taking them, but after a few days the first signals of an attack start again. She feels that the E.Coli shown on the tests at the time she saw me have not fully responded to the antibiotics. In searching for any ways to reduce the acceptance and harbouring of E.Coli by her internal skin, I have made further suggestions:

1 Eat natural yoghurt from her local health food store. A Surgeon Captain Cleave, now dead, did much research on E.Coli in the intestines amongst servicemen abroad, and showed clearly in his results that gut E.Coli can be reduced with a daily intake of yoghurt.

2 Bicarbonate of soda removes excess acidity in bladder urine, helping to remove this natural habitat of E.Coli. Gillian is going to take a level teaspoonful every night in water for one month. She says that mornings are always worse, indicating high rates of overnight acidity.

3 With a raw and E.Coli-prone vagina, she is going to soothe it with a twice-weekly or even once-daily douche of bicarbonate and warm water.

On hygiene, Gillian reckons she is now perfect, and this is why she believes that the E.Coli is coming from a descending situation rather than the ascending situation caused by poor hygiene.

Hormonally, her GP is refusing to cooperate on evaluation or any replacement therapy. This is a brick wall.

Backgrounds of heavy antibiotics and possible lowered hormone levels will not help internal skin to throw off bacterial infestation. Why can't doctors see this?

Gillian and James have had intercourse this month, using the sheath, and there have been no side-effects or soreness following these sessions. This has to be some good news.

Follow-up – mid-January

All is deep gloom and I have spent two hours in wide-ranging thought. Gillian is living on antibiotics and has been since 1981. At the end of each course she goes only 48 hours before her kidneys once again ache and the urine burns. Urinary and vaginal cultures are showing excessive E.Coli and other bacterial infections.

The improved hygiene since seeing me will be holding off external rising infections now, but obviously E.Coli has a massive hold internally. Her vision is often blurred, temperatures flare up, she vomits sometimes, her back aches and she shakes. She really has renal pyelitis.

Only when actually on antibiotics does all this stop; but one must ask, should she continue to take these drugs for an indefinite number of years? Of course not! Alternative ideas, investigations, experiments must be made.

Let's have a résumé:

1   The Lippes Loop coil insertion coincided with the infections beginning.

2   All that time, anyway, she would have been adding E.Coli daily because of her poor hygiene, reference the coil string.

3   Despite all the operations, drugs and urological tests, nothing has worked.

It would appear that my suggestions in the last telephone follow-up have not, in fact, been done. Gillian probably couldn't be bothered, preferring instead to eat the antibiotics. It also probably means that, without admitting to it, she is losing heart and faith in anything working. She's looking for the magic wand that doesn't exist and feels as though a bad fairy has wrapped her from head to toes in a big black cloud. I have spent two lengthy periods of time on the phone with her putting the case for:

1   Joining a health-insurance company. It appears that, through James's job, WPA – mentioned elsewhere in this book, offers him and his family members a 33 per cent discount. They are going to take out a policy.

2   Seeing a proctologist. This is an expert specialist in disorders of the bowel. Just for theory's sake – supposing that the Lippes Loop coil OR the hysterectomy itself (performed, I know, after the start of infections but before the hygiene revision) had minutely damaged the wall of the bowel or intestines allowing a 'leak' of its bacteria? A proctologist might be able to find out, and it's worth at least an investigation in such pressing circumstances.

3   Experimenting at home on another idea which is: referring back to the work and books of the now deceased Surgeon Captain Cleave on the saccharine disease. This is all about modern disorders – like gastric, peptic and duodenal ulcers; dental decay; diabetes; obesity; coronary disease; varicose veins; haemorrhoids; gall-bladder inflammations; constipation *and* E.Coli infestations of the gut! – largely due to modern man's willingness to eat white flour and sugar, and also eating more than you really need.

He says: *A factor in the production of excess acidity by the body is the eating of white flour and sugar. Over-acid urine encourages E.Coli to reproduce.*

He says: *Remove the white flour and sugar and you remove acidity!*

Gillian now tells me that she has had digestive problems all her life, and we know from her notes that she had varicose veins stripped at the early age of 21.

I wonder whether E.Coli, once having been introduced to Gillian's acid system by poor hygiene and the coil string, found a very enjoyable environment from which they refuse to be ejected. Although on first glance she doesn't appear to eat a lot of white flour or sugar, one casserole thickened with white flour might be enough, with other similar daily intakes, to maintain the acidity levels.

It makes health sense, financial sense and medical sense to:

1 Fast for three days: water only, a glassful every one or two hours. Cymalon as described on the packet to further reduce acidity levels.

2 After the fast, slowly introduce brown bread, freshly boiled vegetables, fresh fruit, potatoes boiled with their skins, pears and, a little later, thin slices of medium-cooked meat. No tinned foods or white flour, sugar or artificially sweetened foods.

3 Not much of these foods, either.

By shrinking the fleshy linings of the gut, intestines and bowels, reducing the amount of products for absorption and elimination, we may manage to deplete the food supply and environment for E.Coli.

Theoretically this makes sense and would be agreeable to experts in holistic, homoeopathic or naturopathic medicine. Since other forms of medicine have so far failed, doctors, too, should find nothing to object to in such an experiment. It's cheap to try, faster on results than hospitalization, and less wearing than continuous antibiotics. It may take more than a week – Gillian is in a real state having put on a stone in weight since the hysterectomy anyway, and now probably lacks the willpower to see the experiment through. Just to get her system back in balance after three years of solid antibiotics could take three to six months, even if she packs herself with vitamins and minerals – never mind getting rid of the E.Coli itself.

Practically, will she manage it? Will her willpower reserves stand firm against the demands for her attention and time within the family home?

Two days later

Gillian rang me to thank me for sending the book by Surgeon Captain Cleave. She has read it through avidly, thinks it makes great sense and has totted up roughly the amount of sugar and white flour in her week's normal diet and finds that, indeed, it is a great deal!

She has accordingly decided to take action and is prepared for it to take some weeks to clear her system.

She also has the forms from two insurance companies and is reading them through carefully.

I mentioned the hormones again, and after discussion she has decided to refer back to the gynaecologist who did the hysterectomy to quiz him about hormone therapy, but doesn't feel that he'll be very amenable. As far as I was concerned, the most exciting thing about the phone call was her admittance that she's not 100 per cent on the hygiene. The reason she gave for not always washing, even after coming to me for counselling is that:

1 her house has a separate lavatory next to the bathroom.
2 she can't always get into the bathroom to wash after passing a stool because the family is hogging it!

These points inspired more questions:

Q   When do you pass a stool?
A   Always in the morning between 8 and 8.30.
Q   Since the family leave the house at 8.30 to go their various ways, why can't you wait till they've gone?
A   Because my bowels *have* to be emptied when they want to be emptied and they won't wait!
Q   Do your bowels move in response to eating breakfast?
A   Yes, exactly so.
Q   To allow for an empty house and an empty bathroom, why don't you eat breakfast *after* the family has left?
A   I could easily do that – what a brainwave!

Gillian doesn't go to work, and by delaying her bowel movement she would be able to do the full bottle-washing method in peace and quiet.

Much patience is still needed, but I was extremely interested to hear that her hygiene had remained faulty even after counselling. It would most definitely account for the positive E.Coli and strep reports on her urine cultures and vaginal swabs.

Urine tests will now be of vital interest because if the infections clear we will know why. If symptoms sporadically arise but are minus the named infections, the hormone-replacement therapy will become more desirable; so will lowering acidity levels, which she knows are high but which she now understands and is trying to reduce.

This was a surprising and very exciting phone call.

Follow-up – March

Gillian sent off the WPA form, duly completed and stating that she has a history of urinary-tract infections. It is five weeks since the form was sent back and tomorrow she will phone to enquire whether they have received it.

Since January, the GP has taken one urine specimen and one vaginal swab, both of which were negative – the first for years. She is, however, still being given lengthy courses of antibiotics, which never completely remove the pain in the bladder. After a short break of 4–10 days following a course, the pain becomes unbearable, eyesight blurs over and she's put back on another course. Throughout the last two years this pattern has been repeated constantly, with tests coming back positive – now the first one is negative. A blood test in January failed to show evidence of any blood-borne infections, which is excellent elimination news.

So the hygiene is at last consistent and, therefore, working. But, like so many women, she is misguidedly committed to the idea that the bladder is responsible for this continuing pain and she can't accept that maybe something else, somewhere else in her body, is having a spin-off of symptoms to the bladder.

She is up against yet another wretched GP, who won't even start her on a simple course of hormone treatment for a few months to note any improvements. I expect that unspeakable man is happily dishing out hormones to women patients for contraceptive purposes. Gillian was once on the Pill and had no ill effects, why can't she go on a hormone preparation now? It's scandalous!

If such treatment does not seem to help after a few months – so, well and good, it's another line of enquiry eliminated. At least it won't remove her uterus and one ovary, will it?

Gillian has lost half a stone in weight since adhering to the no-sugar, no-flour routine – this is good news, too, alongside the latest test results.

As soon as WPA accepts her request to take out health insurance with them we may manage to get some private or alternative hormone investigations underway. This would not contravene any possible refusal by WPA to pay for treatment of urinary-tract problems.

Gillian's current symptoms are: back pain, groin ache, bouts of blurred vision, bladder ache, burning urine – no infections either in the urine, the vagina or the bloodstream.

Follow-up – April

I left Gillian a good four weeks before this follow-up to give her time for action. In the event she has felt too depressed and ill to take any action at all, except to telephone the menopause clinic thirty miles away, to be told that they insist on a referral letter from the GP. He won't give one. She also rang a private clinic specializing in HRT, and they also insist on a letter from the GP. Gillian got in a muddle about the WPA form, which certainly requires a medical signature, but only that of the treating doctor – not a signature from the GP as well.

Having put that right, and on more pushing from me, she has rung the gynaecologist who performed the hysterectomy and has an early appointment with him. Prior to my pushing:

1 No further urine or vaginal tests have been undertaken since February, *yet the GP is insisting that antibiotics are continuously taken.*

2 Symptoms are steady of urinary burning, back pain, exhaustion, dry vagina, soreness along the perineum, pain in the groin, bouts of dizziness.

3 Hygiene is now perfect; she washes without fail after a stool.

4 The GP absolutely refuses to refer her anywhere.

5 In despair, the diet has disappeared and weight is being regained.

6 Gillian can't stand up for herself in front of this GP. Five

weeks ago, James went with her to the surgery, only to be told, 'Your wife has a personality problem'!

This general practitioner is wrecking his patient's life. He ought to be helping her to grasp at any straw and research any remote cause for her ill health. I have pushed, pulled, encouraged, advised and sworn – to no avail. And I have flatly told Gillian that she'll remain ill and on needless antibiotics till she's 80!

The coil started it, the ineffective hygiene acting with the coil encouraged rising vaginal infections, and the needless hysterectomy has brought new hormone problems; so after all that the GP decides that his best course of action now is to mimic the ostrich!

Gillian's heartrending cry of 'my hands are tied, I suppose, until I totally collapse' will rattle round in my brain for a long time, making me very angry.

This poor woman is only 35 and could be made well, were it not for red tape, a wicked GP, a lack of drive and a lack of money. Her only asset is me, and she doesn't fully know it because of the years of obeisance to modern medicine. I've done all that I possibly can and I am frustrated and furious about this woman's suffering and imbecilic doctors.

She is to visit the gynaecologist, but only after intense pressure from me. The gynaecologist – who, in my opinion, performed the needless hysterectomy and does not, therefore, have my greatest trust! – has agreed to see her without a referral letter and is willing to do a blood test to assess the hormone situation. He will also work on the WPA form so that Gillian will not foot any bill.

If nothing comes out of the visit to him, Gillian is agreeable, now that she has the funding, to come to London, where one of my experts will start work on her.

I must stress that this woman is one, I suspect, of hundreds of thousands of women from John o' Groats to Land's End also struggling with the red tape and uninformed doctoring that is so haughtily prevalent.

In simple finance and expense, the tranquillizers, antibiotics and needless operations for cystitis and associated conditions which don't make the patient well must be regarded as a waste of government (electorate's) money. To stick so rigidly to outdated investigations and ideas is repressive and retrogressive.

We must seriously question the teaching units in our big hospitals which are still promoting the same old treatments for this commonest and costliest of women's ailments.

We must question the system which insists that a patient stays with one general practitioner and does not allow that patient to move on elsewhere when it can be seen to be a necessity. Vets are competitive – one is free to choose where one takes one's animals for help: one can choose one's dentist and leave; one can choose one's solicitor. This rigid GP system must be discussed afresh at government level.

We must question the patient's blind acceptance of the doctor as being infallible. Somehow the patient must be persuaded that it is all right to query a treatment or investigation, and somehow we must make each patient more knowledgeable.

How one can hope to achieve any of these points, bearing in mind the great spectrum of human nature, is truly beyond me, and even I bow to the reality of a hopeless situation.

CHAPTER SEVENTEEN

Tracy and Zoe Sears

It was Grandma Sears who contacted me. Her letter about her two grandchildren dropped through the letter-box one Saturday morning, and because they lived in my parents' home town, I combined two visits. I spent an hour in the Sears' company, and took lunch later with my parents.

Three generations of Sears gathered in the cosy living room of a warm, modern, semi-detached house on a little development of similar designs in roads variously entitled Honey Close, Broome Avenue, Lavender Grove, and so on. The dog, a white smooth-haired terrier, had an acute affection-seeking syndrome manifesting alternately as a prone body baring its stomach or leaping up and down wrecking your stockings with an unwholesome lust for attention! The room was full of sunshine and autumn dried-flower arrangements surviving for ever the vain efforts of the gas fire to dehydrate them.

Fortified with tea and warmth, for the day outside was crisp, I settled back in the patterned brown velvet armchair facing the three ladies Sears; the fourth, Tracy, aged seven, was at school. Her younger sister Zoe aged four, was not at playgroup this morning. Zoe was straight out of the mail-order catalogues: two big brown bunches of hair, erect at the roots and secured with elastic, hung right down to her shoulders, flickering round the jumper. Lacy white tights peeped out from a little pleated skirt and disappeared into a clean pair of brown sandals. A poppet she was, as she perched on Grandma or on Mum or on the dog!

Mum wore tight jeans, high heels and a sweater, and had short straight brown hair. Attractive but without make-up, she was friendly and smiling and very keen to learn. She has never read anything about cystitis; she had never needed to.

Grandma Sears, on the other hand, had read about it – her sources being my first book and any magazine article coming her way. She herself had been a lifelong victim. From 'knowing' her husband at 16 during an air raid down the garden shelter, right through to his sad death in 1980, she had been dogged by attacks all those years. Her husband had cradled her tear-stained face many a time in their bathroom and had compassionately shared each attack of cystitis with her by comforting and caring. Obviously they had adored one another and had kept a happy home, into which their sons brought their future wives. All the daughters-in-law have a very happy in-law relationship and Grandma Sears is not only part of the scenery in her children's homes but is a great confidante and carer for the younger womenfolk.

Grandma Sears wasn't my microscope material, but it was fascinating to know that she was a victim, that her daughter-in-law had never ever had any problems, but that the two grandchildren had both inherited the predisposition/sensitivity through her via her own son.

I never thought to ask if he was a sensitive, prone-to-poor-health type of person.

If such an inheritance link is ever traceable, my feelings are that it is in some way a skin/membranous sensitivity. As you will see, in comparing some of the grandmother's routines with some of those of the daughter-in-law, the life-style proved dissimilar. For example they use different soaps.

Cystitis is still very under-researched. One of the many aims of this book is to stimulate a few bright specialists to push a few more boundaries, and the aspect of hereditary skin-sensitivity as a factor is just one requiring more work.

Here were three generations. The daughter-in-law flouted every rule in the book, including wearing jeans, and never had a twinge in her life; the mother-in-law took every advice, tip and prescription, and was scourged; and now the grandchildren, currently not taking advice, had already required medical intervention and at an early age knew what their own mother did not – pain and discomfort.

What was it all about?

Tracy, aged 7 years

She had her first attack of bacterial cystitis, minus the bleeding, thank heavens, in January 1983. In the previous September she had started school down the road at the infants' section, so cystitis began after only one term at school. Two further attacks occurred during 1983. She has had one attack in 1984 – in April.

Symptoms are: a red bottom (perineum), frequency, burning urine and an aching tummy.

Urological history

Each attack has shown infection (so the doctor says) in the mid-stream urine results, but he has never named it/them.

Antibiotics were prescribed and Ceporex seemed the most efficient. Two ultra-sound scans of the kidneys have been taken. The first showed one kidney slightly smaller, but six months later the second one showed that both were now level in growth.

There is no refluxing ureter.

All blood tests are normal.

General health

Tracy has excellent health and is very lively.

Hobbies

Mucking about! Riding bicycles, playing with friends, swimming most Sunday afternoons in the local public pool.

Habits

Tracy usually passes a stool AFTER her nightly bath. She and Zoe share the bath, into which they liberally pour the current bubble-bath. I viewed a large, half-empty and highly poisonous-looking bottle of purple liquid without one named constituent. The girls have been using bubble-baths since Tracy was a toddler. Hair is washed in the bath once a week with Johnson's baby shampoo. No grown-up sits in their hair shampoo; why do we let children do so?

Palmolive soap is used as the household soap. Grandma uses Pears. Palmolive is used all along the perineum at bathtime each night.

Underwear is all-cotton, not nylon. It's white and washed with the general laundry.

Woolly tights are worn in winter.

Mum has just bought both girls their first jeans, and as yet they have not worn them.

When Tracy passes urine she wipes with toilet paper but, as Mum says, 'reaches all the way underneath and pulls the paper up to the front!'

My suggestions

1 Ask Tracy if she ever does number two at school.

2 I showed all three ladies the bottle-washing method upstairs and told them how, why and when it should be done. Tracy will be allowed to choose a plastic bottle, as against the heavier glass bottle, which she could drop and cut herself.

3 No bubble-baths ever again. Let her scream her protests, but don't give in. Bubble-baths can start soreness into which bacteria will move.

4 Don't wash Tracy's hair in the bath, wash it over the bath with the hand shower and give her a dry towel for her eyes.

5 Palmolive is not good for sensitive skins. Change to Simple Soap, and even so don't use it anywhere else on the perineum except the back passage. The front part is far too sensitive.

6 Teach Tracy to put appropriate amounts of loo paper onto the loo seat at school before she sits on it.

7 No chemicals of any sort should touch her bottom.

8 Teach her to dab dry after passing urine, not reach and pull.

9 Revise her procedure for using loo paper after passing a stool to make sure that the paper doesn't touch any further forward.

10 Make sure that she is having enough drinks at school.

11 Jeans rub. Don't ever let her wear any.

12 Tracy is obviously very sensitive. Everything in her present and future life-style is important for preventing urinary-tract discomfort.

13 Chlorination of swimming pools is a known cystitis aggravant. Check in future for this as a possible trigger.

14 Following the basic principles, check up and think of everything, with my books as a guide, if another attack starts.

Zoe, aged 4 years

Symptoms

Bouts of burning urine and sore bottoms. First bout – November 1983 during the first term at playgroup. The second bout was at the start of the November 1984 term. A 'scanty' infection was found in the second MSU and Zoe was given five days of antibiotics. It was this particular bout that prompted Grandma to write to me.

Urological history

None.

Hobbies

Same as Tracy – generally mucking about. Playgroup is every Tuesday and Friday morning. There are 29 toddlers, and two lavatories which pass inspection with flying colours at any time – the lavatories pass inspection, I mean!

Habits

Grandma and Mum both say that, like most little girls, Zoe 'holds it'. So does Tracy, and they jig up and down instead of doing what they should do. Zoe doesn't seem to me to drink as much as others of her age, but Grandma thinks it's probably enough. There is rather too much orange squash featuring. From early morning till bedtime only orange squash is drunk. Twice a week at playgroup Zoe has a few sips of milk with the mid-morning biscuits. When she goes to Grandma, she drinks grapefruit juice because Grandma thinks the vitamin C is good for her. All the bubble-bath, hair shampoo, soap and swimming factors are the same as for Tracy. The sisters share much of their life, food fads included, and Zoe will eat a banana every day and possibly more.

My suggestions

1   Halve the amount of orange squash. Substitute milk or water. At four years old, she's probably not ready to like weak tea yet.

2   When her urine burns and her bottom gets red, Zoe must be cajoled into drinking lots more water and therefore 'pressured' into passing it.

3   Fruit juices are too strong for the system of such a small child.

4   No more bubble-baths, they are dreadfully bad for women and girls and should be labelled like cigarettes with a government health warning.

5   Four bananas a week is enough – no more.

6   Watch for any pattern to attacks. None has emerged as yet, but with Mum now enlightened she might spot something. Hopefully my visit will prevent further trouble.

7   Give Zoe a full Disprin if and when another bout of burning urine starts. Crush it in jam and have lots of liquid to drink.

8   Alkalize that burning urine with a half-teaspoonful of bicarbonate of soda in jam, followed again by a good drink.

My comments

Tracy and Zoe are typical cystitis children. Basic medical tests as with Tracy are negative. Therefore we look to the life-style habits and sensitivity. There aren't enough past attacks to give sufficient clues, but now that Mum and Grandma are better informed they can both keep a good watch on the girls.

Tracy was chronologically first with symptoms. It began in January 1983, Zoe's began in the November term of playgroup 1983. The 'unknown' infection could have been pus cells finally resulting from a non-bacterial source like the bubble-bath. On the other hand it could well have been an E.Coli. Tracy's habit of passing a stool *after* the bath and having faecal contamination for the whole of the next day until bathtime combines with her habit of pulling lavatory paper forward every time she passes urine. However, this may have caused all or none or some of those four attacks. The fact remains that such hygiene actions probably ought to have caused more.

I strongly suspect the bubble-bath, the bananas, cold weather, the Palmolive soap and the swimming for the bouts of burning skin and urine.

Once a week their sensitive skin will be immersed for 20 or 30 minutes in a chemically contaminated bath of shampoo, bubble-bath and Palmolive. Several times a week two of those products are present.

In cold weather, as with grown-ups, little girls' kidneys are 'excited' and manufacture more urine. When the bladder, on this impulse, expels urine that lost liquid must be replaced by drinking and by coming indoors to warm up. This will counteract the stimulus of the cold and chill. Little girls dancing around and 'holding it' because they are busy playing a good game will just increase the bladder stress. From the dates, we see that most of the girls' urinary discomfort has occurred in cold or chilly weather.

Mum and Grandma watched carefully as I demonstrated the bottle-washing procedure upstairs. The bathroom has a bath, basin, lavatory and bath shower. Both basin taps can be reached easily while sitting on the lavatory, so the bottle method is simple for them.

We can't really follow up Tracy and Zoe, though I daresay Grandma will do so, and now that Mum is alerted there may hopefully be no further recurrence for either child. With only three bouts between them this year, albeit the latest very recently, it may be many months before another one happens and I can't hold up the book indefinitely.

Suffice it to say that the case history of these two little girls has been opportune for those women dealing with a similar situation in their own lives.

We'll regard the three generations as being 'armed for combat' but aiming for a 'negotiated peace'!

Follow-up – July

Both girls got through the Autumn, Winter and Spring without a recurrence of any symptoms. Mum and the GP are well pleased and put the success down to self-help.

Grandma Sears is much relieved and puts the success down to a 17p first class stamp!

Conclusion

If one thing is striking about all these women, and indeed the hundreds of others that I have seen to date, it is that they should have needed to see *me* at all! Who is to blame for all this suffering?

Can one honestly accuse the medical profession and hold them entirely responsible? I don't think so. They aren't given courses in modern life-styles; urologists aren't taught to regard cystitis and other urinary symptoms as anything other than a urological phenomenon, and GPs simply cannot, with such heavy workloads, fully understand the minutiae of every illness that science has uncovered.

Nevertheless, since cystitis is so common, they could contemplate and rewrite their basic investigative rules for patients coming to them with early attacks of cystitis and regular cystitis. They might run thus:

1   Carefully take urine specimens and TELL THE PATIENT THE RESULT.

2   Pass the patient a leaflet describing the bottle-washing process or the titles of my other books, published by Arrow Books.

3   Always check the state of the vagina and if in any doubt refer to the best gynaecologist dealing in disorders of a difficult or obscure nature.

4   Again use a leaflet or the above books, pointing out the emergency routine for alleviating the early symptoms of an actual attack of cystitis.

5   Prescribe a short course of antibiotics ONLY when an infection of the urine is *proved* present AND the attack is already heavily established.

6   If necessary, after many attacks, order an IVP, but if specimens

show E.Coli or other faecal material don't bother – talk about hygiene.

7 Listen to the clues that the patient drops during consultation and don't scoff at her. Her life-style may well be responsible and only she knows how she treats her body within that life-style.

8 Don't keep a closed mind; continue to learn and don't hide behind the 'urethral syndrome' with a shrug of your shoulders.

9 Work on prevention of cystitis because prescribing yet another course of antibiotics denotes failure to find the cause(s) of her problem.

Can we hold the patients entirely responsible for their adversities? We can certainly hold 80 per cent of them responsible for their own cystitis but we can't *blame* them for being thus so. Women have in one sense to go backwards in time for answers and in another sense must move forward to balance the enjoyments of modern life with the more constrained restrictions essential for good health.

This involves learning – and learning, on such a massive scale the world over, takes time. If one isn't receiving the necessary teaching from older women, then my books and occasional 'correct' media items become learning resources. To learn from other female contemporaries is still unsatisfactory – they may have incorrect knowledge. I suppose what we are endeavouring to achieve is a revolution in health attitudes.

I don't regard this as 'alternative' medicine. It's true that I'm offering other alternatives than just more antibiotics for cystitis patients and their doctors, but my alternatives aren't fashionable, and they do still work well within conventional scientific medicine. Self-help is no more, no less than plain common sense.

Thrush is not dealt with in quite the same manner. Here I fully agree with what the medical profession prescribes for treatment and the fact that they don't refer on anywhere. That's all quite acceptable and I can offer no further suggestions except to extol the virtues of the VD units, but my efforts are 100 per cent on prevention which can *only* be practised by the patient.

In a further comment, whilst applauding the medical profession for their treatment of thrush, I should accuse many of them of irresponsibly prescribing heavy and prolonged courses of antibiotics which do cause so much modern thrush. Short, sharp courses are better, cheaper, and should be combined with additional advice on thrush prevention via my books. I do find that more and more doctors are adopting this short-course idea, and it certainly lessens side-effects of all sorts.

Although this latest book contains only 17 patients who came for counselling, I think that valuable points arise on every page from which we can all learn. Apart from the obvious practicalities and solutions, it becomes provocative. I set out to be one thing and one thing only – a detective. Detectives experience a range of emotions – anger, elation, frustration, satisfaction, disappointment and, the worst of all, acknowledgement of failure. I certainly never fail completely with any patient; that they learn and practise correct care of their genito-urinary systems at home and avoid infections is triumph. In others, removing aggravating secondary causes will aid the unmasking of the real cause, and yet more cases can be prevented from worsening. I often have complete successes in women who have previously trekked everywhere for help. Unhappily, some returned to their own areas where poor interest and lack of appropriate medical facilities will render investigations virtually impossible; and there are also those women – one of them is illustrated in this book – who for all manner of excuses and reasons won't be taking advantage of the help that I have mapped out for them.

There may be doctors who will happily pick holes in this book, but let them not forget that their kind probably had the initial failures without which their patients would not have needed to visit me.

Victims has been described to me as 'riveting' – it is also, dare I say it myself, sensational. For an unlettered patient to counsel on a medical illness pushing known treatments and investigations, criticizing and commending – this is the stuff of history. Few patients have such colossal cheek, but I do it with a very real sense of righteousness and a sense of message. Not only am I completely well now and have been since 1971–2, but so are millions of women all over the world, either directly from the books or from reprint articles in huge national newspapers or from the countless TV and radio shows which promoted my message. This active record replaces grand letters after my name, and tucked inside the righteousness is a very real humility at being given the gifts to get the message across and give so many women the chance to get well.

There was a Hungarian doctor in the nineteenth century called

Semmelweiss. He fought his own kind all his life just to promote the virtues of washing hands before attempting to deliver a woman in childbirth. He showed many times over that this simple procedure stopped childbirth fever from killing his own patients. His peers and contemporaries scoffed and scorned and refused to recognize him or his hygiene. He ended his days in a lunatic asylum from the pressures and rejection.

I have certainly not suffered so, and I take comfort and encouragement from that man's example. I hope you may feel that the cases in this book prove it.

Glossary of Terms

Anaemia   low level of iron in the blood
Anus   opening for passage of faeces
Artery   blood vessel carrying blood *from* the heart
Bacteria   germs
Bicarbonate of soda   baking soda, an alkalizing agent
Bladder   elastic sac in the pelvic region which stores urine
Candida   thrush; a fungus infection of the mouth, vagina and
   rectum
Catheterization   insertion of a small tube to withdraw urine from the
   bladder
Cauterization   burning away of infected skin
Cervicitis   any inflammation of the cervix
Cervix   neck of the womb
Colitis   inflammation of the colon (part of the bowel)
Cystoscopy   an operation for investigation of the bladder
Diabetes   illness caused by lack of insulin in the bloodstream
Dialysis   artificial cleansing of the blood by a machine
Dilatation/dilation   enlargement of cervix or urethra by the insertion
   of rods
Distal urethral stenosis   condition of the bladder during menopause
   or old age
Diuretic   an agent which stimulates the production of urine
Diverticulitis   inflammation of the bowel
Diverticulum   small false bladder growth
E. coli   natural bacteria which inhabit the bowel
Enuresis   bed wetting
Episiotomy   an operation on the perineum during difficult childbirth
Epithelium   skin

Foreskin   skin covering the end of the penis

Fungus   growth of detrimental yeast organisms

Gonadotrophin   hormone involved in ovulation

Hexachlorophine   an antiseptic used frequently in hospitals

Hormone   a chemical messenger carrying instructions from glands to organs

Hormone imbalance   incorrect balance of hormones

Hysterectomy   removal of all or part of the internal female sexual organs

IVP   intravenous pyelogram, or kidney X-ray

Labia (majora/minora)   folds of skin which protect urethral and vaginal orifices

Litmus paper   chemical papers able to test for acidity/alkalinity

MSU   mid-stream urine specimen

Menopause   natural process involving termination of menstruation

Micturition   act of passing urine

Micturating cystogram   an X-ray taken during urination

Monilia   thrush; a fungus infection of the mouth, rectum and vagina

Oestrogen   hormone involved in ovulation

Ovulation   release of unfertilized female egg from the ovaries

Perineum   base of the body's trunk containing excretory orifices

Pituitary gland   chief sexual gland of the brain responsible for most hormone activity

Potassium citrate   alkalizing agent

Prostate gland   male sexual gland through which passes the urethra

Pyelitis   kidney disease

Radiographer   specialist in X-ray techniques

Rectum   tube for passage of stools to the outside

Reflux   urine flow in the wrong direction

Renal scarring   scarring of the kidney by constant disease

Sphincter valve   valve attached to the sphincter muscles controlling output of urine

Streptococcus   a form of bacteria

Trichomonas   sexually transmitted disease

Ureters   tubes carrying urine from the kidneys to the bladder

Urethra   tube carrying urine from the bladder

Urethral syndrome   medically unaccountable symptoms of cystitis without bacteria

Urologist   doctor specializing in renal organs

Uterus   womb
Vagina   birth canal
Vaginal thrush   milky, irritative discharge from the vagina
Vaginitis   any inflammation of the vagina
Vein   blood vessel carrying blood *to* the heart

NOTES

NOTES

NOTES